apple cider vinegar for health and beauty

apple cider vinegar for health and beauty

Recipes for Weight Loss, Clear Skin, Superior Health, and Much More—the Natural Way

Simone McGrath

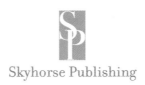

Skyhorse Publishing

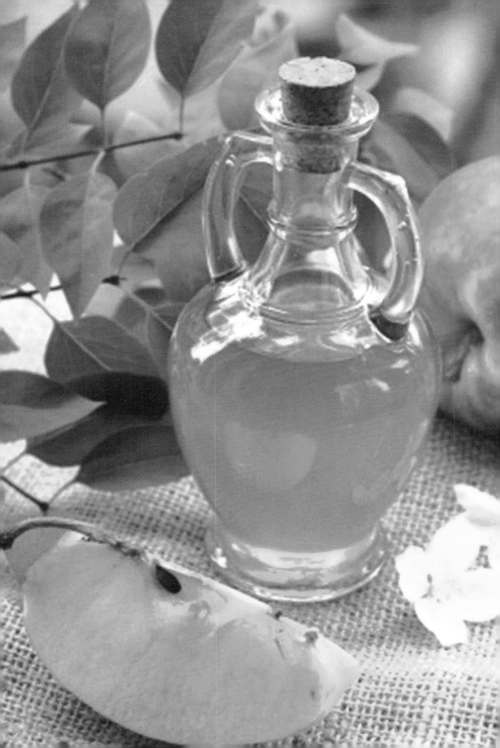

Skyhorse Publishing books may be purchased in bulk at special discounts for sales promotion, corporate gifts, fund-raising, or educational purposes. Special editions can also be created to specifications. For details, contact the Special Sales Department, Skyhorse Publishing, 307 West 36th Street, 11th Floor, New York, NY 10018 or info@skyhorsepublishing.com. Skyhorse® and Skyhorse Publishing® are registered trademarks of Skyhorse Publishing, Inc.®, a Delaware corporation.

www.skyhorsepublishing.com

10 9 8 7 6 5 4 3 2 1

Library of Congress Cataloging-in-Publication Data is available on file.

Print ISBN: 978-1-63220-693-0
Ebook ISBN: 978-1-63220-954-2

Printed in the United States of America

contents

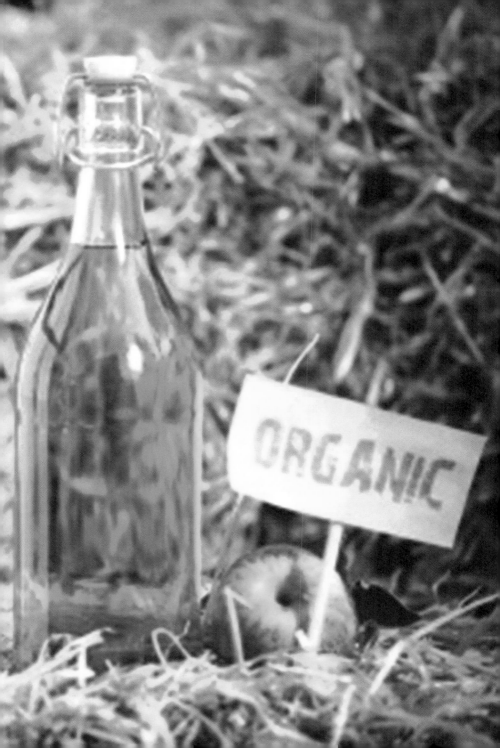

Introduction

Look out honey, there's a new kid in town! That's right folks, honey is not the only amber liquid that can boost health, healing, and vitality. There is another amber liquid that is worth its proverbial weight in gold. This lesser-known phenomenon has recently taken the world by storm and is fast becoming a household name. Its remarkable benefits are responsible for health gurus, nutritionists, and doctors alike singing its praises, and it is being heralded as "nature's finest healer."

Ladies and gentlemen, allow me to introduce apple cider vinegar!

Health, weight loss, fat burning, beauty, and restoration are just some of the qualities contained in apple cider vinegar's impressive and ever-expanding résumé. It can be used to revitalize your home, and not even the loyal family dog is exempt from enjoying the benefits of this wonderful liquid, as it is a natural flea repellant!

Legend has it that in an effort to win a wager with Mark Antony that she could spend a fortune on a single meal, Cleopatra dissolved a pearl in a glass of vinegar and drank the costly cocktail. Whether this tale is true or not we will never know, but the fact is that the exceptional power of apple cider vinegar is nothing new. Its virtues have been extolled through the ages from as early as 5,000 BC when the Babylonians used it as a condiment and preservative, and long before Cleopatra drank her expensive concoction, Hippocrates was using the tart liquid for its incredible medicinal qualities. In fact, it may well be one of humankind's earliest recorded remedies.

Over the centuries, vinegar itself has been fermented from an impressive number of different products, including fruits and berries, coconuts, beer, potatoes, and honey, to name a few. Vinegar is actually an incredibly versatile product that can be derived from many sources. As has already been stated, any fruit can ferment into vinegar, but vinegar can also be made from many different types of grains, the most common being rice. Rice wine vinegar is incredibly popular in Asian cuisine and is enjoyed the world over. In fact, vinegar is so versatile that it can even be made from wood chips. Yes, you read right.

However, when creating vinegar from grains or wood chips, the starches contained in these products first need to be converted to sugars. Once this has taken place, the fermentation process can start.

But no matter what product is chosen as the base for vinegar, by far the most endearing of all is the vinegar made from apple cider. It will take something truly spectacular to oust apple cider vinegar as the darling of all natural remedies.

So read on and find out exactly why this amazing amber liquid has got everyone talking!

Let's get the nitty-gritty science facts out of the way first.

Along with yogurt, cheese, beer, and wine, vinegar is one of the most popular foods created from yeasts and bacteria. Most vinegar is created from fruit juice when it is exposed to yeast and bacteria, which react to the sugars in the juice in different ways. The yeast ferments the sugars, causing a chemical reaction that changes it to alcohol, then the alcohol is further broken down into acetic acid by specific bacteria. Acetic acid is the base component of vinegar. The yeasts and bacteria that break down fruit sugars into vinegar are commonly found in nature, which explains why, when the juices are extracted from fruits, they naturally progress through the stages of fermentation and acetification. Now while this process sounds less than appealing, I think we can all agree that the end products are simply divine.

The family of bacteria that are responsible for converting alcohol into vinegar are called acetobacters. What is interesting is that this particular family of bacteria has been at the center of heated debates amongst scientists who disagree on how many types of this bacteria actually exist. This means that isolating a pure strain of this mysterious bacteria for vinegar-making can be considered as much a science as an art.

When alcohol changes into vinegar, the chemical reaction results in a substance called cellulose. This fibrous substance can easily be seen in homemade vinegar or in a bottle of wine that has turned to vinegar. This thick filmy substance floats in the vinegar, often near the top, and is called the "mother of vinegar." The mother is often erroneously believed to be respon- sible for creating vinegar, but it is actually the end result of the whole process rather than the initiator. However, as the "mother of vinegar" is likely to have a large concentration of acetobac- ters clinging to it, it can successfully be used to introduce these organisms into cider, for example. Acetobacters also occur abun- dantly in our natural environment, but need oxygen in order to grow and survive. When alcoholic beverages like apple cider are exposed to the air for a period of time, the interaction between the acetobacters and the oxygen facilitates the process of converting the alcohol into vinegar, and the result is apple cider vinegar.

As the cider is transformed into vinegar, the alcohol content of the liquid drops and the acidity levels rise. The best and easiest way to determine when the acetification process is complete is to taste the liquid. There should not be any odor or flavor of alcohol present. The strength of the final vinegar product is dependent on the amount of alcohol in the original cider. Most of the vinegar that is used in the average household measures around 4 to 6 percent acidity, and the alcohol content of the apple cider should be around that percentage too.

The natural tendency of fruit juice to ferment is perhaps the reason why alcoholic beverages and all kinds of vinegar have featured so prominently in the diets of almost every culture in the world, and still remain staples in many regions today.

The word "vinegar" is derived from the French term *vinaigre*, which literally means "sour wine" (*vin* meaning "wine" and *aigre* meaning "sour").

Apple cider vinegar is without a doubt one of the healthiest things you can take for maintaining good health. It can be incorporated into almost any aspect of your daily routine, from your meals, to smoothies, to simply taking a spoonful or two every morning. It doesn't matter what your preferred method of consumption is, just so long as you take it. Trust me, in a few weeks you will be reaping the rewards of this amazing elixir!

So congratulations on taking the first step to good health. This book will become your apple cider vinegar bible and will help you learn everything there is to know about this incredible liquid and all it has to offer you.

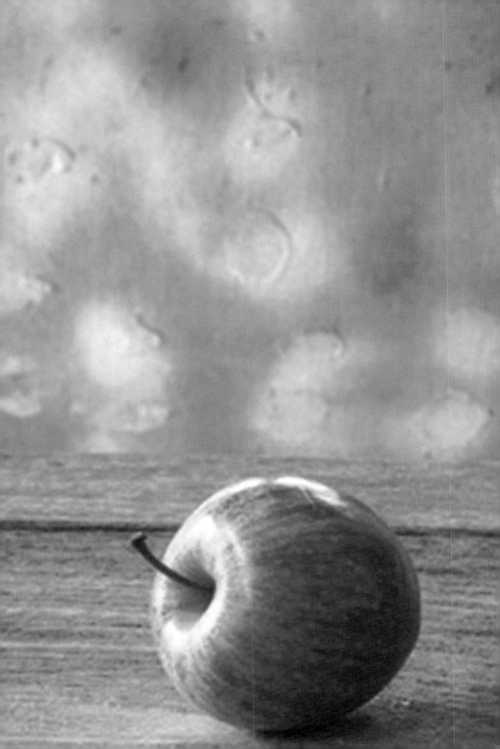

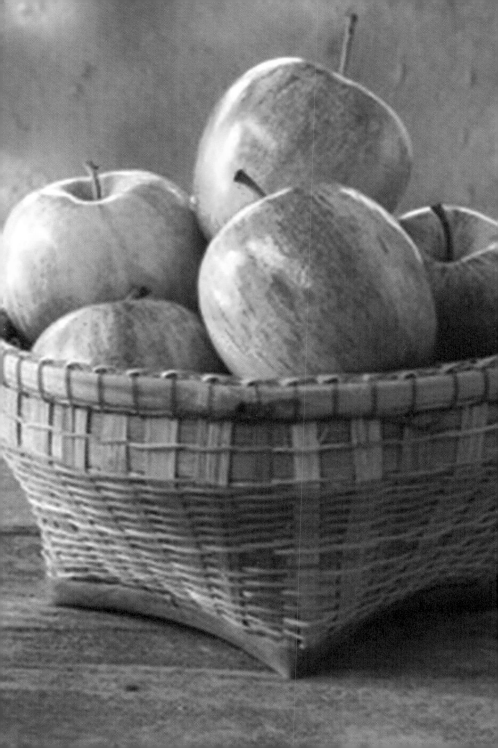

How to Make Apple Cider Vinegar

While there are plenty of wonderful pre-made brands of organic apple cider vinegar available in health shops, there is something intrinsically rewarding and satisfying about making your own.

Here is an easy to follow step-by-step process for making apple cider vinegar:

1. Find a wide-mouthed container that will hold a sufficient volume of liquid for you. (The wide mouth is so that there is sufficient surface area to facilitate oxygen absorption.)
2. Sterilize the container and then fill it to two-thirds full with hard apple cider.
3. You now need to add a little unpasteurized and unfiltered apple cider vinegar—this will still have live bacteria in it. Alternatively you need to add some "mother of vinegar," which you will be able to buy from most health shops or brewing stores.
4. Put the container in a dry, clean, dark, out-of-the-way area that is stable in temperature and cover the top with a cheesecloth. The cheesecloth will allow oxygen in while keeping insects and other contaminants out.
5. Wait for four weeks, and then taste it—yes, you need to taste it! This is the centuries-old foolproof method

to see if the vinegar is ready. You should not be able to taste any alcohol when the process is complete. Alternatively, for those less adventurous souls, you can use a wine testing kit to tell you when the acidity levels reach 5 or 6 percent.

6. Do not be tempted to test the vinegar too soon, and when you do, try to disturb the layer of "mother of vinegar" as little as possible. Some of the bacteria may sink to the bottom of the container when disturbed and decompose, which will affect the taste of the vinegar.

7. When the apple cider vinegar is ready, you can strain it through a paper coffee filter to remove the "mother of vinegar" or you can carefully remove it using a fine mesh spoon or a large serving spoon. Either way keep some of the vinegar with some bacteria in it to start your next batch.

You can also make apple cider vinegar from whole apples, it just takes a little longer.

1. You need two glass bowls, one larger than the other, and as many apples as will fill the larger bowl.

2. Wash and quarter the apples, then place them in the larger bowl. Leave them to brown and then fill the bowl with water until the apples are covered. Cover the bowl with the apples in it with a cheesecloth and leave it in a warm, dark, and clean place for six months.

3. When the six months is over, you will notice a grayish scummy film on top of the water. This means that the process has been successful.

4. Now strain the liquid from the bowl through a coffee filter into the second bowl. Cover the bowl again with cheesecloth and leave it in the same place as before for another four to six weeks.

5. When the apple cider vinegar is ready you can strain it through a paper coffee filter again to remove the "mother of vinegar," or you can carefully remove it using a fine mesh spoon or a large serving spoon.

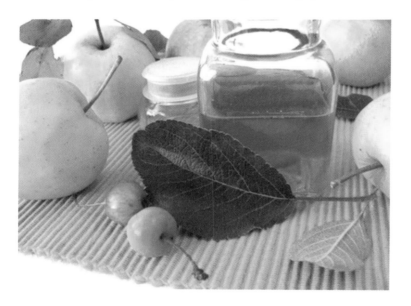

Commercially, the producers of vinegars have tried to hasten the above processes and increase the volume of batches by using many inventive means. With what has become known as the Orleans method or the field process, manufacturers, originally in France and now most commercial cider vinegar producers in the world, use fifty-gallon wooden barrels filled to half capacity and laid on their sides to maximize the surface area exposed to air. Holes, covered in mesh to keep contaminants out, are usually drilled in each end to aid airflow. The manufacturers also need to speed up the fermentation process, so they do this by adding an oxygenating substance such as wood chips or corncobs to the barrel.

In 1823 the German, or fast method, was developed for making vinegars. With this method fermentation takes place in a tower packed with charcoal, corncobs, and wood shavings. The cider or wine is trickled into the top of it and air is fed in through the bottom. The result of all of this is vinegar in weeks, not months.

Even Louis Pasteur, the famous French scientist, got involved in improving the production and quality of vinegar. In 1858, he invented a wooden raft that would float on the surface of the vinegar and stop the "mother of vinegar" from sinking to the bottom. He also wrote extensively on the bacteriological processes involved in the making of vinegar thus improving the understanding of what affected the quality of the product.

The most modern method of producing vinegars is the submerged tank method, which uses a man-made "mother of vinegar" called acetozym. The vinegar produced by this method, however, is dead, meaning it has the required sharp flavor and acidity characteristic of vinegar, but nothing else. It is precisely the natural fermentation process and the work of the "mother of vinegar" that provides the multitude of health benefits that we seek from this veritable panacea.

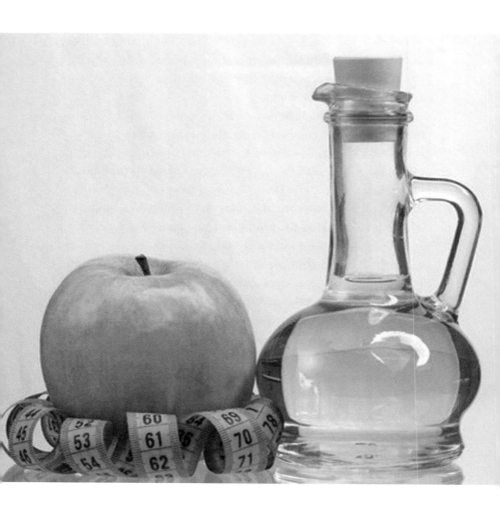

Apple Cider Vinegar Nutrition Facts

Apples are a veritable goldmine of vitamins, minerals, and nutrients. They pack a powerful nutritional punch and are truly deserving of the age-old adage, "An apple a day keeps the doctor away." These powerhouses contain beta carotene (an antioxidant), pectin (a soluble fiber), as well as a host of minerals, the most notable being potassium. One apple contains 10 percent of your recommended daily allowance of potassium! Quite amazing for such a small and unassuming fruit!

Unfortunately, it is quite sad that generally a clear vinegar is regarded as more aesthetically pleasing and accordingly, to meet consumer demand, the manufacturers comply with societal pressure and end up filtering and pasteurizing the vinegar they produce. This means that the "mother of vinegar" is removed as along with any sediment. This process stops the activity of the acetobacter bacteria, the precise thing that makes the vinegar nutritionally effective. These live cultures are responsible for the complexity of flavors present in the final product and renders the vinegar full of character by injecting the liquid with its healthful qualities. So while you may end up with a product that is commercially acceptable because it can be regulated the world over, you are essentially compromising many of the vital qualities that make it so effective for good health.

The high quality vinegar that Dr. Jarvis wrote about in his book, *Folk Medicine*, in which he espoused the use of a daily dose of apple cider vinegar and honey, can today be found in Braggs Apple Cider Vinegar. Braggs Apple Cider Vinegar is unpasteurized, unheated, and unfiltered and contains all the wonderful health promoting qualities and nutrition of the apples from which it was made.

One only has to examine the following list of nutrients below to recognize the immense potential in apples and apple cider vinegar.

1 MEDIUM APPLE (100g)

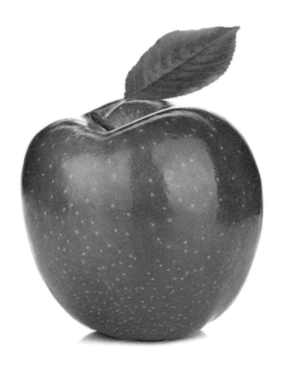

Calcium	6 mg
Energy	218 kJ
Carbohydrates	13.81 g
Dietary Fiber	2.4 g
Fat	0.17 g
Protein	0.26 g
Folate (B9)	3 ug
Iron	0.25 mg
Magnesium	5 mg
Manganese	0.035 mg
Niacin	0.091 mg
Pantothenic	0.061 mg
Phosphorus	11 mg
Potassium	107 mg
Sodium	1 mg
Vitamin B1	0.017 mg
Vitamin B2	0.026 mg
Vitamin B6	0.041 mg
Vitamin C	4.6 mg
Water	85.56 g
Zinc	0.04 mg

1 TABLESPOON OF APPLE CIDER VINEGAR (15g)

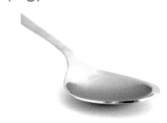

Calcium	1 mg
Calories	2
Iron	0.1 mg
Phosphorus	1 mg
Potassium	15 mg
Water	14.1 g

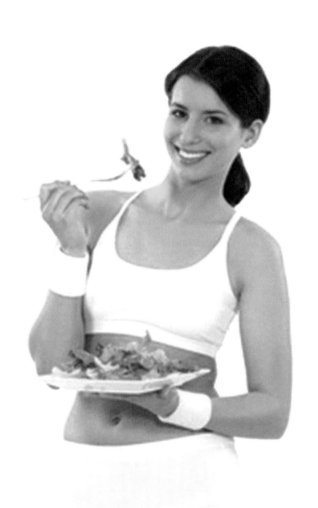
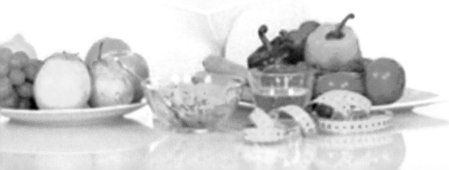

Losing Weight with Apple Cider Vinegar

Apple cider vinegar can be the basis of an effective weight loss strategy: FACT!

In order to convince any doubters out there, let me give you some of the facts about fat, the role it plays in our body, and how we go about eliminating it. If you can garner a basic understanding of these processes, it will become clear to you exactly how apple cider vinegar can work to aid the body's natural processes and help you to lose those excess pounds. Apple cider vinegar is natural—it's not a medicine and it's not a drug, nor is it some miracle fat burner or diet pill that promises the earth and then leaves you wanting. What it is, is a supplement—a natural remedy that you can take every day. Even if you don't believe all the claims, take it anyway and let the results speak for themselves.

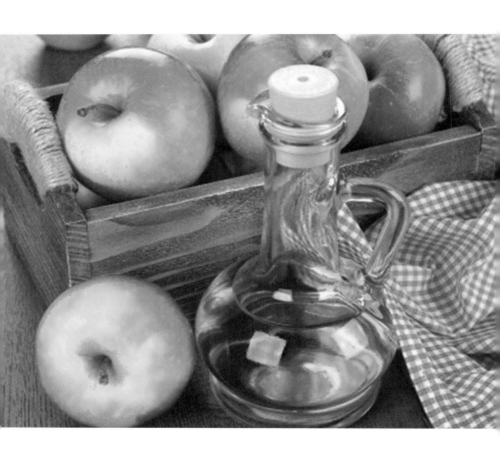

How Does Fat Affect Us?

Fat plays a critical role in keeping our bodies healthy and functioning at their best. Now wait, that is not your golden ticket to run off and scarf down a box of donuts! We need only a certain amount of the *right kind* of fat in our diets, whether we are watching our weight or not. But granted, getting this right is nothing short of an incredibly delicate balancing act, especially when there is so much contradictory literature on the subject out there. But don't worry folks, I am here now to lay out the no-holds-barred truth about fat and what it does and doesn't do for our bodies, with the hopes that it will help all of you develop a healthier relationship with the dreaded leper that we all do our best to avoid!

So welcome fat back into your lives folks, but do so cautiously!

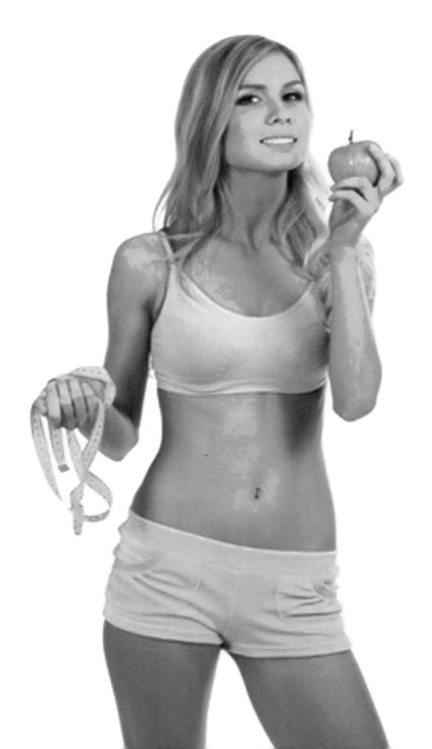

What Does Fat Do For Our Bodies?

Sometimes in order to give the right answer, we first have to ask the question in the right way. To properly answer the above question, we have to answer two questions:

1. What purpose does storing fat in our bodies have?
2. What external and internal factors affect the usage of fat?

The most critical reason for our bodies to store fat is to provide us with a storehouse of fuel. This portable resource is there to see us through periods where food is scarce or temporarily unavailable. Our bodies have evolved and adapted over thousands of years to survive harsh winters and long migratory treks as hunter gatherers. They have also needed to provide us with energy on demand to hunt when we haven't had a meal for a period. Life was pretty rough and brutal back then so our internal organs needed "shock absorbers" to allow our vital organs to survive heavy impacts from falls and blows from our prey. We thus have deep body fat around our livers, lungs, heart, and other organs.

In modern society food is readily available all year round, however our bodies are still driven by our biological imperatives. Funny how our resolve to stick to our diets and eating plans crumbles close to Christmas. The decrease in daylight as winter approaches is a trigger for our bodies to store more fat, to insulate us, and see us through the lean winter months. However, our bodies are amazing biological machines that make our modern lifestyle possible. When we eat, our bodies burn the carbohydrates for instant energy and the protein is also used as a fuel source, but it is our stored fat that that gets us through the long haul of work and exercise.

There are various internal and external factors that affect the way our bodies store and utilize fat. We also need to differentiate between the different types of ingested fats, such as saturated and unsaturated fats and what they do to and for our bodies. These categories of fats are broken down further into many sub-groups, mono-saturated and poly-unsaturated fats are some examples of these.

The major factor in where our bodies store fat is gender. Males tend to start storing fat on their tummies and then spread it evenly over the buttocks, legs, chest, arms, and back. Females tend to store fat mostly on their buttocks, hips, and chest, and then evenly over the rest of their bodies. This difference is again thanks to evolution and Mother Nature!

The interaction of the fats and the other food we ingest with our bodies is greatly affected by the health of our bodies. And in turn, the health of our bodies is greatly affected by the foods we ingest and in what quantities and ratios we ingest them. This is because of the many different types of fat in the food we eat and the fact that these different types of fat react differently with our bodies. If your digestive system is not healthy it can compromise its ability to digest and extract sufficient amounts of the nutrients we need. It is this relationship between food and health that apple cider vinegar interacts with and aids.

During the digestive process, most of the fats we eat are absorbed by our bodies and then recombined and used in the various chemical reactions taking place in our bodies. Certain fats are involved in the reaction of enzymes in the body, some aid the activity of hormones, some vitamins such as A, D, E, and K require the presence of fat in order to be absorbed. Fats also play a role in the health of our nervous system. When combined with the mineral phosphorus, they produce lecithin. Lecithin is required for the production of neurotransmitter chemicals and these chemicals help the brain regulate appetite, mood, and cognitive functions. Some of the fats the body requires cannot be reconstituted, such as Omega-3 and Omega-6. Omega-3 and Omega-6 are fatty acids that work in opposition to one another, so getting the correct ratio in your diet is essential. Omega-6 aids the active responses of the body, raises blood pressure, and aids clotting and cell regeneration. Omega-3 does the opposite and aids the "calming responses." These fatty acids can be found in various foods such as fish, green leafy vegetables, wheat germ, and olive oil to name a few.

Generally speaking, it's the ratio of saturated to unsaturated fats that we have to watch in our diets to maintain long-term health. Unsaturated fats are beneficial to our health, while too much saturated fats are detrimental. While both occur in a variety of foods, studies show that they do not occur in equal quantities. Unfortunately, saturated fats are far more prevalent in our normal diets than unsaturated fats. Saturated fats are found in processed foods and animal products such as dairy products, meats, pastries, and chips. Unsaturated fats are found in foods such as nuts, olives, and avocados. The chemical structure of saturated fats is saturated with hydrogen atoms and contains no double bonds between carbon atoms; they are generally not liquid at room temperature. Unsaturated fats have double bonds in their chemical structure, have less hydrogen atoms, and they are generally liquid at room temperature.

So, as you can see, the right amount of the right kind of fats is vital in order to keep our body functioning at its best. There are many ways in which apple cider vinegar helps us to make the best use of the fats we consume in order to improve health and promote weight loss, but more about this later. Let's take a look at the ways that fat works in the body—for better or for worse.

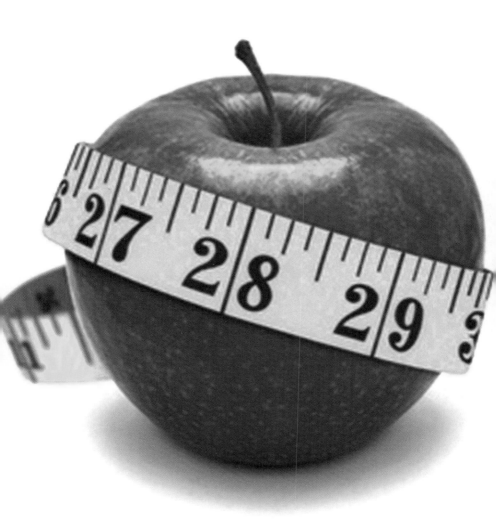

How Does Fat Make Us Fat?

Its elementary dear readers: If you consume the same or less calories that your body needs to function, you will never get fat! Now I am not going to launch into a good and bad food lecture, because we all know what we should or shouldn't be eating. Ladies, you know you are going to regret inhaling that whole slab of chocolate as you sit and watch *Friends* reruns, and guys, you know that you shouldn't be eating a double burger, fries with cheese sauce, and a liter of soda as you watch your favorite sports game.

It is pretty clear to all of us that being in good shape has a marked effect on our quality of life. Carrying extra fat increases your chances of disease and chronic health issues such as infertility, arthritis, stroke, kidney disease, diabetes, heart disease, and cancers of the prostate, breast, stomach, and colon, to name a few!

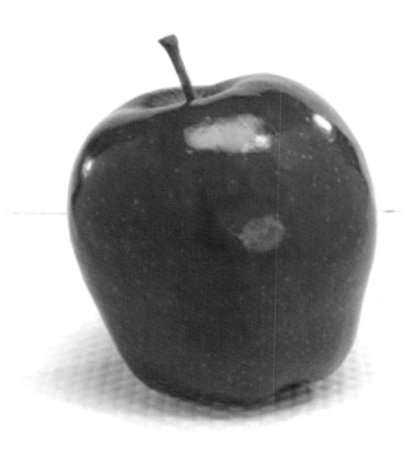
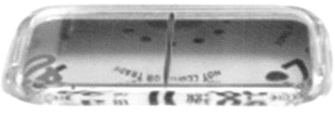

How Does the Body Process and Eliminate Fat?

There are many different mechanisms at work in the body that determine how much fat the body uses. It is very difficult to lose fat or stay slim if even one of our mechanisms is not functioning properly. Our metabolism, the overall rate of activity in our bodies, is one of the most important mechanisms. It is affected by our genetic makeup, our weight, the amount of exercise we do, our body fat percentage, our body temperature, how much sleep we are getting, how well our thyroid is functioning, what we eat, our age, and our gender.

In terms of our genetic makeup it seems that some people's bodies tend to store fat more readily than others. The theory some have put forward is that there is a "thrifty gene" in some people. This "thrifty gene" is what would have allowed some of our ancestors to survive cyclical harsher winters. They would have stored more fat than most other people, so when a particularly barren winter or other natural disaster occurred, the individuals with this gene would have stood a better chance of survival.

Our weight, or our lean body mass, is another factor that affects how much fat we burn. The more muscle mass an individual has the higher the energy requirements to "run" the body (big cars use more fuel). Thus, tall, larger framed people's bodies require more energy to keep going day to day than small, slightly built people.

People who exercise for long periods or who have a lot of muscle mass will burn off the food they take in relatively quickly and the body then turns to its fat stores for energy. Bodybuilders eat six to eight meals a day to maintain their size and provide their bodies with enough resources. This is so they don't burn muscle mass when their fat stores are depleted. Long-distance runners and professional cyclists need to take in food when competing. This is because their body fat percentages are already so low.

People with a high body fat percentage more than likely lead a sedentary lifestyle. Their bodies will more than likely get all their energy requirements from the food they eat and still have some leftover to store as fat. There are, however, other factors that have an effect on body fat. The "set point theory" concept is that your body has a stable quantity of fat cells by the time you are an adult. The more weight you carried in your childhood and your teenage years, the more fat cells you will have as an adult. These fat cells then become "fuller" or "thinner" as you gain and lose weight as an adult. The set point is the trigger in these cells that will send a message to your brain saying that your fat cells are getting too thin and that you must eat more. Different people's fat cells will have different set points, and the strength of the message is affected by the number of cells. Thus a person with lots of fat cells and a high set point will battle with cravings for food when dieting.

The set point in the cells is affected by their sensitivity to insulin. The byproduct of the breakdown of most of the foods we eat is a simple sugar called glucose. As the level of glucose in your blood rises, your pancreas needs to start secreting more insulin to unlock your cells, so that they can use it for energy. If your blood sugar is constantly high from over-eating and not enough exercise, your insulin levels will also be high. This can lead to a condition known as insulin insensitivity. When this happens your cells don't react to the insulin in your blood and therefore don't allow the glucose into your cells to be burnt as energy along with the fat. It is very hard to lose fat with this condition. This is one of the main causes of adult diabetes.

When the insulin in our blood reaches the receptors in the fat cells, it tells them to allow glucose in. When the glucose enters the fat cells, it reacts with the fat and oxygen from our blood to give off energy that our bodies can use. Heat is a byproduct of this reaction and the faster the rate of the reaction, the more heat is given off. This is called thermogenesis. People with a high rate of reaction are therefore burning more fat than those with a low rate of reaction. The rate of thermogenesis will naturally vary from person to person, but a low rate can also be caused by insulin insensitivity. Again, dietary health and a lack of exercise play a role.

Diets high in fats and refined carbohydrates combined with a lack of exercise wreak havoc on our body's blood sugar regulating mechanisms. These factors lead to insulin insensitivity and eventually diabetes. When a person becomes obese from over-eating, their blood glucose will be high and this leads to diabetes. Diabetes hinders the body's ability to burn glucose and fat, which leads to obesity.

There are ways to counteract insulin insensitivity and improve thermogenesis and thereby reduce the amount of fat we carry. The pillars of this are diet and exercise. So called slow release carbohydrates, such as vegetables and fresh fruit along with legumes and whole grains, are good sources of soluble fiber and release glucose into the bloodstream more gradually than refined foods. Exercise helps reduce the glucose level in the blood by thermogenesis and the rate of thermogenesis will improve as the fat cells become more sensitive to insulin. Exercise will therefore improve the effectiveness of a good diet, and the more you exercise, the better the results will be from doing it.

How much sleep we get and a regular sleeping pattern can also play a role in fat loss. The pituitary gland releases a growth hormone which is a protein-based peptide hormone. This hormone stimulates growth, cell reproduction, and regeneration in humans. These functions require energy and thus a healthy release of this hormone has a secondary benefit of burning energy while we sleep. Nearly 50 percent of the human growth hormone release occurs during the third and fourth REM sleep stages. Studies have shown that a healthy diet and a regular sleeping pattern aid the amount and consistency of human growth hormone release.

There is a reason why we crave sweets and starches when we diet. Tryptophan is an amino acid that is released into the brain when we eat. While the brain is receiving regular doses of tryptophan it determines that we are getting enough to eat. If the levels of tryptophan become low, the brain thinks starvation might be imminent and stimulates the urge (craving) to eat. We crave carbohydrates because they provide a quick energy release and a quick release of tryptophan. Constant dieting or fasting can create an imbalance in tryptophan and eventually lead to binging.

Having a good source of fiber in your diet will also help you regulate your weight. As well as improving your insulin sensitivity, fiber helps you feel fuller and reduces the number of calories your body will absorb. An example of a water-soluble fiber is pectin. Anybody who has made jam or jelly at home knows how pectin congeals when mixed with water. This has a positive effect on weight loss because the same thing happens with water and pectin in your stomach. It therefore makes you feel full for longer. Apples have a high level of pectin and can improve your chances of effective weight loss by helping to curb your appetite.

High-fat-content meals generally leave you feeling full for longer because fats are most often among the last nutrients to be absorbed in the digestion process. It is important, as I've said before, to eat the right kinds of fats in the correct ratios. There is also a smart time to eat your fats. If you tend to battle with cravings in the afternoon or just before bed, try having more fats with your lunch. Adding some walnuts or having an avocado with your meals will help curb those cravings and keep them under control. If you can't climb into bed without raiding the refrigerator, try having a large salad with olive oil and apple cider vinegar dressing with your dinner.

Diets high in salt can lead to water retention, and although being overweight is primarily as a result of carrying too much fat, water retention can also leave you feeling bloated and lethargic. If you ingest too much salt or your diet lacks potassium it can lead to similar symptoms. Potassium acts in the opposite way to sodium in our bodies. Where sodium helps our cells retain water, potassium helps them eliminate it. Thus, adding substances with a high potassium content, such as apple cider vinegar, can help balance the amount of water in our cells. Lowering your salt intake along with this is still the best course of action for optimal results.

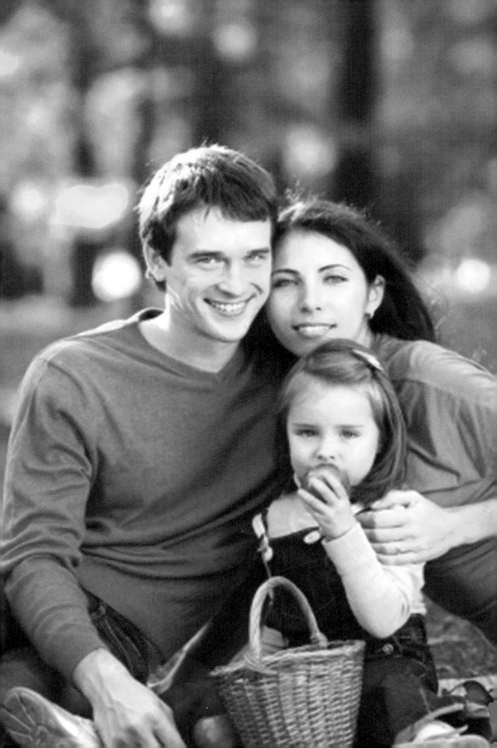

Staying Healthy With Apple Cider Vinegar

Good health, to a certain degree, is achieved and maintained in the human body when there is equilibrium or balance between all the various substances that affect and take part in the reactions that keep us alive.

The cells in our bodies are constantly exchanging fluids. The rate of exchange, the volume of exchange, and the direction of the flow is a result of how salty these fluids are. The various organs in our body also depend on the specific acidity and alkalinity of different substances in order to perform their functions properly.

Apple cider vinegar is able to benefit our health because of its effectiveness in being able to balance these acids and alkalines, along with helping to maintain the equilibrium between fluids and salts.

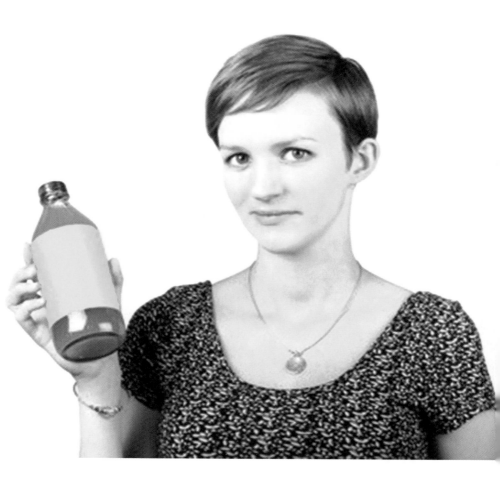

Getting to Grips with the Acid/Alkaline Balance

Whether a substance is an acid or an alkaline base is one of its most basic properties. In most reactions and processes that occur in animals and plants, acids and alkalines are formed to balance each other out.

Many physicians and nutrition researchers promote theories related in some way to the acid/alkaline balance in our bodies. The foremost of these being Elson Hass along with James Balch and his wife Phyllis Balch. However, although they all agree that the acid/alkaline balance is very important to maintaining good health, they do not agree on whether the human body's natural/best state is to be slightly acid or slightly alkaline. Doctor DeForest Clinton (D.C.) Jarvis, who was practicing medicine more than a hundred years ago, was particularly interested in the acid/alkaline balance in the human body and how apple cider vinegar was able to help achieve such a balance.

The basic premise of the acid/alkaline theory states that when foods are ingested and metabolized in our bodies they create either an acid or an alkaline ash. The pH measurement or the level of acidity or alkalinity of the ash does not necessarily correspond to whether the food itself is considered highly acidic or not. An example of this is lemons; they are acidic when we eat them but the ash they leave behind after being digested is alkaline. Diets high in refined carbohydrates, wheat, fats, and meat are considered to increase the body's acidity. In this state the human body is more susceptible to illness and many chronic ailments such as frequent colds, infections, congestion, and migraines. Alkaline-producing foods include fruits and vegetables, but since most people eating a western diet tend to eat too few of these, the problem of over-acidity is much more prevalent than over-alkalinity.

Acids are not all bad though; they are essential for digestion. Hydrochloric acid combines with enzymes in our stomachs to break down protein in the foods we eat. As we age, we tend towards producing less hydrochloric acid than we need to digest proteins completely. It is thought that getting indigestion might be as much a problem of having too little stomach acid as having too much. This is why it is suggested that you take a little apple cider vinegar before you eat. The apple cider vinegar promotes acidity in the stomach and aids digestion, enabling you to obtain all the nutrition available from the food you eat. In addition to this, apple cider vinegar contains tartaric acid and malic acid. These acids deter the growth of disease-promoting bacteria in the digestive tract and also food-borne pathogens, thus promoting good long-term health.

Fruits and vegetables are good sources of minerals such as magnesium, calcium, sodium, and potassium. They are important because they bind with acids and neutralize them. They are therefore an important part of maintaining the acid/alkaline balance of the body at a health-promoting level. Apple cider vinegar can help in maintaining the acid/alkaline level by supplementing our supply of these alkalizing minerals and as has already been noted, it is especially high in potassium.

A healthy acid/alkaline balance is not only important to our digestive system. Vinegar has been used for a very long time in douches as an effective remedy for vaginitis and yeast infections. Apple cider vinegar has also been used as a remedy for many skin problems. This is because the pH of apple cider vinegar is very close to the pH of human skin, in that it tends to be slightly acidic.

Acids also have strong preservative abilities. This is because most bacteria and molds cannot survive in a highly acidic environment. This is why vinegar and other naturally occurring acids have been used through the ages to preserve food. The most widespread examples of this are pickling and canning. Apple cider vinegar is particularly popular for pickling as it adds a delicious fruity flavor to relishes, pickles, and other preserves.

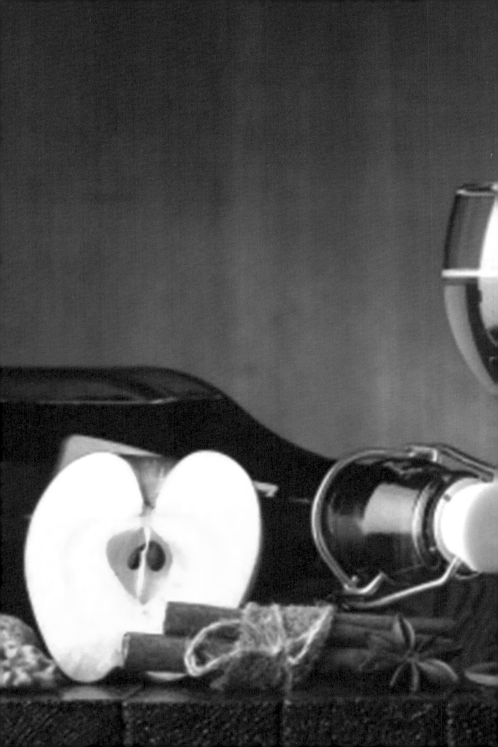

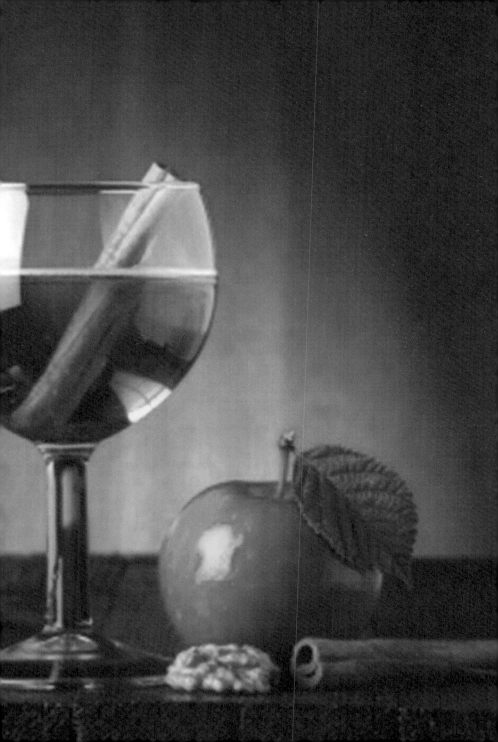

Getting to Grips with the Fluid/Salt Balance

One of the most important equations in the interplay of body chemistry is the relationship between salty fluids and water. It is basic biochemistry that if there is a salty solution on one side of a membrane and water on the other side, the water will be drawn in the direction of the salt solution. This process is known as osmosis. One of the most common examples of this effect is the drying and curing of meat with salt.

Using the same principles, two of the major electrolytes, potassium and sodium salts, perform a balancing act with water on either side of our cell walls. If we had a deficiency of potassium, the sodium solutions outside our cells would draw water out of them and we would eventually dehydrate. Electrolytes act as conductors for our nerves' electrical impulses, which is why dehydrated people lose coordination and have muscle twitches. Water retention is also a symptom of low potassium, rather than too much sodium. Because there is not enough potassium to keep the correct level of water inside our cells, the higher concentration of sodium outside the cells draws the water out of the cells and into the tissues around them. Our skin is the largest body of tissue we have and it then swells from this extra-cellular water. This is what we call bloating. The best course of action a healthy person can take when they experience intermittent bloating, as with menstruation, is to supplement their diet with a little potassium as found in apple cider vinegar. This is far healthier than the drastic, commonly espoused treatment of cutting out salt and overhydrating. This can lead to electrolyte imbalance and negatively affect other vital reactions taking place in our bodies.

Over the thousands of years that our bodies evolved and adapted to the food available in the environment, salt (sodium chloride) was hard to come by. In modern times we enjoy a state of dietary affluence where salt is plentiful. Our body chemistry has, however, not changed. In addition to this, the proportion of leafy greens and fruit in our diets, our source of potassium, has fallen. Besides its role in maintaining our fluid/salt balance, potassium also makes it more difficult for bacteria to get enough moisture from our cells in order to grow and multiply. As potassium works to keep water in our cells, it helps to keep tissues soft and healthy. Potassium also aids kidney function by moving the water in our bodies to them.

Potassium is vital in maintaining a healthy, properly functioning metabolism. This is because it affects the utilization of carbohydrates and proteins. As we get older we unfortunately have a more difficult time extracting and retaining the potassium from our diets. A deficiency in potassium can lead to abnormal or even a lack of cell growth. This often leads to disturbances in heart rhythm, elevated blood sugar, dry skin, muscle weakness, and fatigue. In severe cases, a lack of potassium can lead to changes in the central nervous system, kidney problems, and fragile bones.

Apple cider vinegar is a great source of potassium with 15 mg per tablespoon, as well as containing other important minerals. Another very good reason to include some apple cider vinegar in your daily diet.

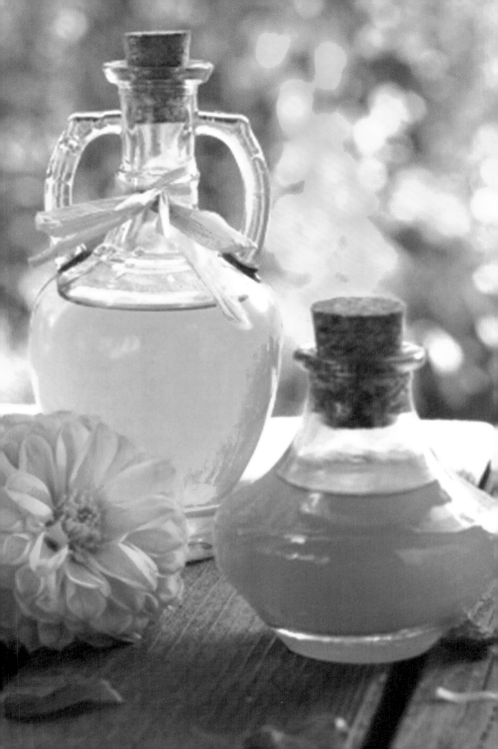

Is Apple Cider Vinegar A Probiotic?

A common misconception about apple cider vinegar is that it is a probiotic, when in fact it is a prebiotic. Prebiotics promote healthy digestion by encouraging and aiding the growth of good bacteria in our guts. Probiotics on the other hand *are* the good bacteria. The key ingredient in apple cider vinegar is the pectin from the apples it is made from. Pectin slows nutrient absorption because it binds to products in our digestive tract that our bodies cannot make use of, such as cholesterol, toxins, pathogens, and harmful bacteria. Once the pectin from the apple cider vinegar binds to the unwanted product, it carries it from our bodies by way of our regular bowel movements. This leaves the probiotics in our digestive systems to grow, flourish and keep us healthy.

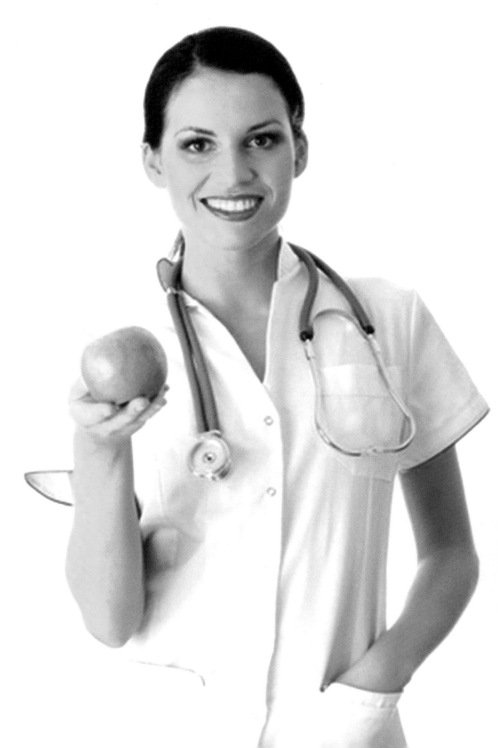

Apple Cider Vinegar—Your Personal Medicine Box

I am sure by now you are coming to the realization that there is something special about this simple liquid—and you are quite right! As one of the earliest recorded remedies, apple cider vinegar has literally stood the test of time as a healer for centuries. Its continued use all these years later is testimony to the amazing qualities and powerful nature inherent in it. Furthermore, apple cider vinegar has held up under modern scientific scrutiny and while, as with anything, there is contention over the finer details, among the experts there is a general consensus in the effectiveness of a simple tonic made with apple cider vinegar. It is recommended to drink this tonic three times a day, preferably before or during meals. If, however, you find that consuming the tonic at mealtimes upsets your stomach, you can try drinking it a little while after your meal. If mealtimes are just not conducive to this because of a busy lifestyle, or perhaps you don't stop your day for the customary three meals a day, you can drink a glass upon waking, one when you are going to bed, and simply mix up this easy formula in a flask or shaker and have it on the go sometime during the course of the day. Whatever works best for you, just so long as you drink it!

So what is this magical concoction?

Apple Cider Vinegar Tonic:

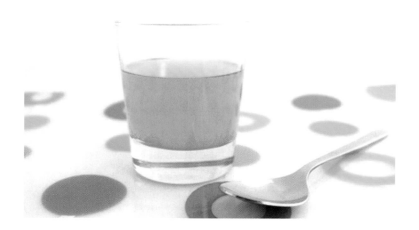

Yields: 1 Serving

Ingredients:

    250 ml water
    1–2 tablespoons apple cider vinegar
    Raw organic honey to taste (optional)

Method:

    Mix the ingredients together in a large glass.
    Sip it at your leisure.
    Feel the difference!

Try this basic formula to start experiencing the benefits of apple cider vinegar. Experiment with the amount of vinegar you add, starting with the least and building up your tolerance over time until you find a level that works for you. As it can be quite a tart taste, you can add a little raw honey to the mixture. And I am sure you have all heard about the wonders of raw honey, so this gives your body a double whammy in health-giving properties! This tonic is better tolerated and more effective if sipped slowly, so use this as your excuse to put your feet up and relax for a few minutes!

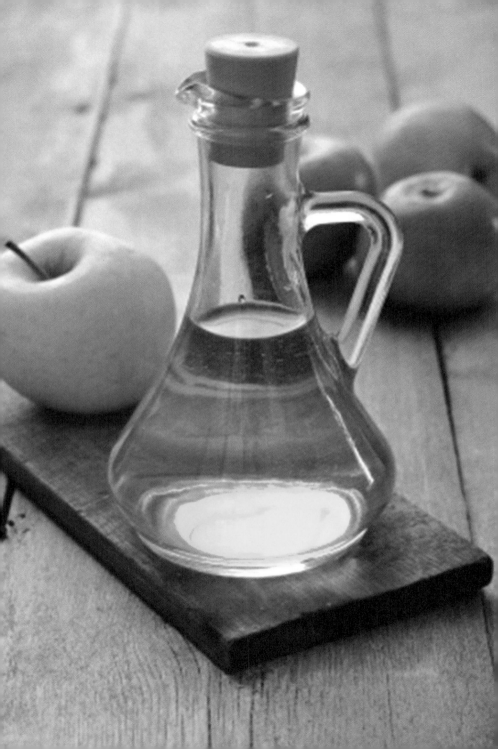

Apple Cider Vinegar for Everyday Common Ailments

In addition to the general tonic for overall health there are many tried and tested folk remedies that use apple cider vinegar for specific conditions and ailments. Here is a compilation of the most common ones that you might find useful.

ACNE - Combine 2 cups of apple cider vinegar with 1 pound of grated horseradish. Allow the mixture to sit for 2 weeks, then strain it through a fine mesh sieve. Use a cotton ball to apply the liquid to the acne spots daily and you will soon see an improvement.

AGE SPOTS - Mix 2 teaspoons of apple cider vinegar with 1 teaspoon of onion juice. Apply this solution to the darkened areas of skin daily and you will see them begin to fade in about 2 weeks.

AGING - Could apple cider vinegar be the elixir of youth we have all been searching for? Seems so. Simply combine 2 teaspoons of honey and 2 teaspoons of apple cider vinegar in a glass of water. Drink this mixture daily to give your metabolism a hearty boost which in turn will restore your youthful radiance. A sluggish metabolism is the death knell for beauty—keep your metabolism revved up and in peak condition to stave off the visible signs of aging.

ALLERGIES - Apple cider vinegar may be one of the best allergy treatments available. It has antibiotic and antihistamine powers that are priceless in our modern world where more and more people are suffering from allergy attacks and allergy-related illnesses. Traditional allergy meds are costly and often make the user feel drowsy, and a whopping 3o percent of people report that they don't believe their allergy medicines are effective! An allergic person's body responds to environmental irritants like dust and pollen abnormally by producing histamines to fight off the intruding particles, but all this histamine in their system actually causes all the classic allergy symptoms.

Taking a natural antihistamine such as apple cider vinegar prevents the production and release of the histamines and consequently quells the allergy symptoms too. That's right, no more swollen, red, itchy, watery eyes, no more uncontrollable sneezing and nasal congestion, no more headaches, asthma, and coughs. And all you have to do is mix 1 tablespoon of apple cider vinegar with 1 tablespoon of honey and 1 tablespoon of lemon juice and drink this three times a day. You will start noticing a marked difference in a few weeks once your body has built up its natural defenses to fight off all types of allergies. The key to curbing allergies is to drink apple cider vinegar regularly—what could be easier?

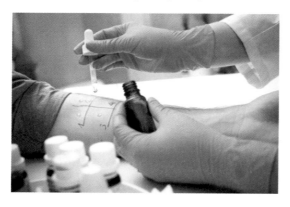

ARTHRITIS - While apple cider vinegar cannot cure arthritis, it can certainly help to relieve the pain and many people have attested to its effectiveness. The potassium in apple cider vinegar is thought to help prevent the buildup of calcium in the joints, which causes the stiffness and pain. Furthermore, it has been suggested that the painful joints characteristic of arthritis may actually be caused by an accumulation of toxins in the joints. Specifically the pectin in apple cider vinegar helps to absorb the toxins and remove them from the body. Apple cider vinegar is a natural detoxifier and will help to purify your whole body. It is recommended to take a dessert spoonful of apple cider mixed in water at mealtimes for relief from pain.

ASTHMA - Apple cider vinegar has been found to strengthen the lungs and immune system, both of which are imperative for asthma sufferers. Combining apple cider vinegar with honey helps to restore the acid/alkaline balance in the body which helps to stop the wheezing that generally accompanies an asthma attack. Sipping a tincture of 1 tablespoon of apple cider vinegar and 1 teaspoon of honey in half a cup of warm water over the course of thirty minutes will provide relief when you are in distress. If wheezing persists half an hour after finishing the drink, then try another dose, although you are not likely to need one as breathing difficulties should have subsided by then. If the first dose of apple cider vinegar and honey does not work, another tried and tested remedy is to soak two cotton pads in apple cider vinegar and apply them to the insides of your wrists while you sip the second dose. Breathing should be easier after this.

ATHLETE'S FOOT - Soak your feet in a mixture of half apple cider vinegar and half water twice a day until symptoms subside or alternatively apply some apple cider vinegar directly to the affected areas a few times a day and at bedtime for relief.

BLADDER AND KIDNEY INFECTIONS - To soothe symptoms drink 1 cup of the following mixture three times a day: one quart distilled water, two tablespoons fresh or dried corn silk, one teaspoon buckwheat honey, half a teaspoon apple cider vinegar. You can chill it if you like.

BLEEDING - Vinegar has been used by physicians for many centuries to treat wounds and stop bleeding. In line with this practice, Dr. Jarvis researched the effects that apple cider vinegar might have on bleeding and came to the conclusion that the adrenaline-like effects of apple cider vinegar was what helped to coagulate blood and thus stem the flow of blood.

Apple cider vinegar taken as a general tonic is also believed to help a person heal quicker after surgery and if taken regularly before a major operation, it will build up the person's immunity so their healing response will be greater. The only exception to this is intestinal surgery.

For Nosebleeds - Simply soak a ball of cotton wool in some apple cider vinegar and place it into the bleeding nostril. Have the person tilt back their head so that the force of gravity will work to reverse the flow of blood. The coagulating effect of the apple cider vinegar will help to stop the nosebleed much quicker than pinching the bridge of your nose or using a plain cotton ball would.

BLOOD PRESSURE - Apple cider vinegar contains potassium. Potassium helps to balance out the body's sodium levels and thus helps to lower blood pressure. Take the general tonic on a regular basis for long term effective relief from the unpleasantness of high blood pressure. Apple cider vinegar also contains magnesium which helps to relax the walls of the blood vessels, effectively lowering blood pressure.

BODY ODOR - Apple cider vinegar is a natural disinfectant and can be used as a body deodorant because it kills the bacteria and germs that are responsible for the offensive odor. Simply soak a cotton wool ball in undiluted apple cider vinegar and wipe it under your arms once a day to effectively kill any smells. For foot odor, make a mixture of 1 liter water and 1 cup of apple cider vinegar. Soak smelly feet three times a week in this mixture to eliminate the bacteria that are causing the foul odor.

BONE HEALTH - Apple cider vinegar contains important minerals for strong and healthy bones like magnesium, manganese, phosphorus, calcium, and silicon. It also contains the trace mineral boron. Boron works to support the metabolism of calcium and magnesium and elevates the levels of estrogen and testosterone in the body, both of which leads to strong bones. Taking the apple cider tonic regularly will be a good dietary source of these minerals, which will sustain bone mass density and will help ward off degenerative bone diseases like osteoporosis.

BREATHING PROBLEMS - *See asthma*

BRUISES - To reduce the swelling and discoloration that accompanies bruising, simply heat ½ a cup of apple cider vinegar over low heat on the stove and then dissolve 1 teaspoon of salt into it. Apply a compress soaked in the warm liquid to the site of bruising and leave it there for thirty minutes. This stops the bruise from developing and eases the pain from swelling.

BURNS - Apply undiluted apple cider vinegar to the site of the burn. This helps to stop pain and swelling and, in addition, it disinfects the wound at the same time as providing much needed nutrients to the site of trauma to promote healing and cell regeneration. This remedy works on both sunburns as well as minor burns from other sources (like hot appliances or boiling water). Although for sunburns over large areas of skin, a warm bath spiked with apple cider vinegar might be more effective. Contrary to what you would think, pouring vinegar onto the site of a burn does not sting and is not painful—you simply feel a tingling sensation which lets you know that the apple cider vinegar is working its wonderful magic!

CANCER - Apple cider vinegar contains numerous substances that can protect the human body against cancer. Beta carotene is known to be a powerful antioxidant. Antioxidants help fight the effect of free radicals in the body. Free radicals are molecules, atoms, or ions that have an open shell due to having unpaired valence electrons. This causes them to attack cells in the body to try and steal electrons from them. This damages the cells and in turn causes them to become free radicals too. This can lead to a cascading effect where a large number of cells can be damaged. Antioxidants have spare electrons in their shells and are thus able to donate electrons to the free radicals, binding to them, stabilizing or deactivating the free radicals before they can attack our cells.

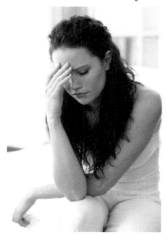

Pectin is found in the skins of apples and in apple cider vinegar, and is a soluble fiber that keeps food from stagnating in the colon. This decreases the amount of toxins released from digested food in the gut by helping the body eliminate it quickly.

Research indicates that having a pH balance in your body that is slightly alkaline is helpful in preventing or slowing down cancers in the body. Some people even state that having an alkaline pH balance has cured them! Apple cider vinegar, although highly acidic, leaves an alkaline ash or residue after being processed by our bodies. This promotes a long-term alkaline pH in our bodies.

Vinegar has also been shown to be very effective in detecting cervical cancer, even better and more cost-effective than pap smears in rural locations. In a study published in *The Lancet* by researchers from Johns Hopkins University in Baltimore and the University of Zimbabwe, nurse-midwives screened almost eleven thousand women by using the VIA method. VIA (direct visualization with acetic acid) is where the nurse or doctor uses a cotton swab to apply acetic acid to the cervix. After thirty to sixty seconds a bright light is shone and the cervix is inspected. Pre-cancerous lesions, which have a higher ratio of intracellular proteins, turn white when combined with acetic acid. Researchers on the study expressed the view that "the vinegar test was more likely to pick up precancerous or cancerous cells than the pap smear."

CANKER SORES - You can relieve the pain of canker sores and speed up the healing process by applying apple cider vinegar directly to the sore with a Q-tip. Do this at least twice a day after eating. This will initially cause some discomfort, but after a few minutes the pain and discomfort will subside. For a less painful method try rinsing your mouth with diluted apple cider vinegar, it will be less painful, but the healing process take longer.

CANDIDA - Candida is a condition where there has been an overgrowth in the normally friendly and necessary Candida Albicans yeast. It occurs naturally in all our mucus membranes and one of its most important functions is to recognize and destroy harmful bacteria. Candida Albicans is, however, not supposed to overgrow and get out of control while we are still living. One of its secondary purposes is to help break down the human body when it dies. Candida Albicans and apple cider vinegar do not get along. Mix a tablespoon of apple cider vinegar with a glass of water and drink it before every meal. The apple cider vinegar actually kills the yeast and therefore helps fight the intestinal overgrowth. For external relief you can add a cup of apple cider vinegar to your bath or use it as a douche by mixing two tablespoons of apple cider vinegar to one quart of warm water. Do this twice a day until symptoms are gone.

CATARACTS - Cataracts are generally the result of damage to the lens of the eye and are a common problem of aging. Studies have indicated that if you have a diet rich in beta carotene and vitamins C and E, all of which are present in apple cider vinegar, you will be less likely to get cataracts. Diets high in salt and fats have been shown to increase the risk of getting cataracts. Taking two tablespoons of apple cider vinegar mixed with water or juice twice a day is the general tonic for optimum protection.

CHICKEN POX - Apple cider vinegar can relieve the discomfort of chicken pox. You can apply full strength apple cider vinegar to the affected areas as well as adding one cup to a warm bath.

CHOLESTEROL - Research indicates that apple cider vinegar can lower cholesterol. In a study published in a foreign medical journal, scientists found that an apple cider vinegar-enhanced diet may increase HDL, the good cholesterol, and reduce levels of triglycerides. Other research conducted on mice has yielded the same results. Pectin, especially apple pectin, has been found to absorb fats and cholesterol and remove them from the body. Pectin is a soluble fiber and is found in apple cider vinegar. Amino acids are also found in apple cider vinegar, they neutralize harmful oxidized LDL, the bad cholesterol.

COLD SORES - Cold sores are extremely painful fluid-filled blisters that can appear on the face, lips, cheeks, nostrils, and even inside the mouth. They are caused by the herpes virus. Apple cider vinegar is one of the oldest and best household remedies, because viruses like the cold sore cannot survive in acidic environments. You can either take a cotton ball soaked in apple cider vinegar and apply it daily for a less painful but slower remedy, or apply it directly with a Q-tip daily for quicker results.

COLDS AND FLU - Apple cider vinegar can be helpful in preventing and treating colds and flu. While it is highly acidic, apple cider vinegar actually helps the body maintain a healthy pH level. This helps prevent and treat colds and flu by stopping germs from getting cozy in your chest and nose. This is because a body which is kept at a healthy, slightly alkalized state is unappealing to germs. Unfortunately, the western diet most of us eat predisposes us to having an acidic pH balance, so it's no wonder we spend the winter months battling germs with sniffles, aches, and pains. Drinking the usual tonic of one to two tablespoons every morning and night, or when cold and flu season starts, will help prevent or diminish the severity of the sickness. If you already have a full blown cold or bout of flu, take the apple cider vinegar anyway. It will help your immune system fight off the germs and give you some extra energy, as well as improving your digestion. If the cold or flu is affecting your nose and sinuses, add a tablespoon of apple cider vinegar to your humidifier and leave it on overnight. Then there is the age-old remedy for chest congestion. Cut a piece of brown paper bag to the shape of your chest and soak it in apple cider vinegar. Sprinkle the side that is going against your chest with ground black pepper and lay it across your chest. Cover it with a towel and keep the cold sufferer warm. Remove after half an hour, repeat daily.

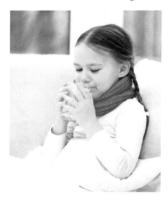

CONSTIPATION - Constipation is usually caused by eating a poor diet too low in fiber. It is also a normal sign of aging as the volume of digestive acids reduces as we age. Constipation can lead to serious health problems because of the increased amount of time digested food remains in the colon. This leads to a greater number of toxins being reabsorbed into the body, leading to free radical damage and a host of secondary illnesses. Eating a diet with a high fiber content is the most effective and natural way of combating and alleviating constipation. Apple cider vinegar is a good source of pectin a water soluble fiber. You can supplement your diet with a daily tonic of apple cider vinegar or you can try a well-known recipe from Patricia Bragg. You need to boil two cups of distilled water and a quarter cup of flaxseed for ten minutes. Then remove it from heat. The mixture will become gelatinous as it cools. You then take a teaspoon of apple cider vinegar and mix it with two tablespoons of the flaxseed gel. Take this mixture every morning and again one hour after dinner.

CORNS - To treat corns, soak your feet in a basin with warm water and a half to a quarter cup of apple cider vinegar, depending on the size of the basin. Remove your feet and dry them. Once dry, rub the corns with a pumice stone. Apply full-strength apple cider vinegar directly to the corn and then cover them with a bandage and leave overnight. Apply more apple cider vinegar in the morning and bandage again. Repeat this process until the corn has disappeared.

COUGHS - Honey is a staple for most coughs and throat ailments; one of the oldest and most common remedies for a cough is a mixture of honey and lemon juice. Apple cider vinegar can be substituted in for the lemon juice. The ideal ratio of the mix is two parts honey for one part apple cider vinegar. You can take anywhere from one teaspoon to one tablespoon of this mixture at a time up to five or six times a day. This mixture is especially good for children who may get an upset tummy from over-the-counter cough medicines. A slightly stronger mixture, more suited to adults but safe for children who can stomach it, is a mixture consisting of: 2 tablespoons apple cider vinegar, 2 tablespoons honey, 2 tablespoons water, a ¼ teaspoon cayenne pepper, and a ¼ teaspoon ground ginger. Place all the ingredients in a jar and shake vigorously to combine. Place the mixture in the refrigerator to store. Shake the jar before usage as the spices will not dissolve.

CRAMPS - Muscle cramps are usually a sign of an electrolyte imbalance such as a deficiency in magnesium and calcium, or a deficiency in vitamin E. Taking a regular daily tonic of apple cider vinegar will supply your body with some of the minerals and vitamins it lacks.

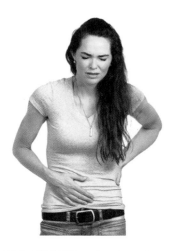

CUTS AND ABRASIONS - Apple cider vinegar has been used for centuries by the armies to treat wounds. Hippocrates espoused its usefulness in healing wounds too. You can apply full strength apple cider vinegar to reduce the chance of infection and also speed up the rate of healing.

DANDRUFF - Recycle an old shampoo bottle and fill it with apple cider vinegar. Apply full-strength apple cider vinegar to your hair and scalp and rub it in. Leave it to soak for half an hour before washing your hair. This will destroy the bacteria or fungus that could be causing your dandruff.

DEPRESSION - Depression can range from serious metabolic disorders to occasional mood problems. The severity and causes can vary widely from individual to individual. Serotonin levels have been found to greatly influence moods. Apple cider vinegar is also believed to help with serotonin levels in the brain. Some Eastern medicine practices subscribe to the belief that depression is caused by having a stagnant liver. Taking a daily dose of apple cider vinegar works as a liver-cleansing tonic. This is promoted by the amino acids that it contains.

DIABETES - Medical research into apple cider vinegar and its health benefits is still very much in its infancy. The area concerning apple cider vinegar's effect on diabetes is one of the most advanced. In many studies it has been shown that apple cider vinegar reduces blood glucose levels. In one study that was published in *Diabetes Care*, the journal for the American Diabetes Association, it was clearly shown that people with Type 2 diabetes who ingested two tablespoons of apple cider vinegar per day had lower levels of blood glucose when tested the following morning. The average level of reduction was measured at four to six percent.

DIAPER RASH - Apple cider vinegar is an effective cure for many forms of rashes due its fungicidal and antibacterial properties. It can be used in a half water, half apple cider vinegar mixture which you dab on with a soaked cotton ball at each diaper change. Another remedy is to mix it half and half with freshly brewed and cooled rooibos/red bush tea, which in itself is an effective diaper rash remedy. This mixture is also applied with a soaked cotton ball at each diaper change.

DIARRHEA - Diarrhea is normally caused by harmful bacteria in the colon or an imbalance in the naturally occurring bacteria there. Apple cider vinegar will not only help the body restore the balance of bacteria in the colon, but the water-soluble fiber pectin will absorb water in the intestine and bulk up the stool. To minimize the stress on the gut, divide up the usual daily dosage of two to four tablespoons into six dosages spread out through the day. If the diarrhea persists for more than two days or the symptoms worsen you must contact your physician as soon as possible.

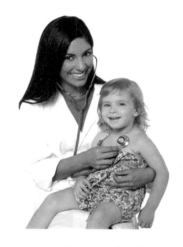

DIGESTION AND BURPING - One of the biggest and most important contributions apple cider vinegar can make to our health and wellbeing is as an aid to our digestive system. It starts as soon as you drink the apple cider vinegar tonic. The acid receptors in your tongue begin stimulating the saliva glands as soon as they come into contact with the apple cider vinegar. Saliva mixes with the food we eat and starts the digestive process, which begins with the breakdown of carbohydrates. Apple cider vinegar also improves the effectiveness of the digestive enzymes and enhances the action of our stomach's hydrochloric acid. Any person who needs to make significant alterations to their diet will most likely be helped by sipping a third of a cup of water mixed with a teaspoon of apple cider vinegar before every meal. Apple cider vinegar's antibacterial properties can also help the digestive acids reduce the opportunity for bacterial infections in the stomach. World travelers might be well-served by taking along a small bottle or buying a small bottle of it in tablet form to take in their suitcases when traveling. Apple cider vinegar can also be effective in lessening the effect of overeating or eating an overly rich meal, or a meal eaten too close to bed time, by speeding up the breakdown of food in the digestive.

DIZZINESS - Dizziness can result from having an overly alkaline condition in the body. There are also a number of conditions that affect the central nervous system by causing conflicting messages from the eyes, ears, etc., to be sent to the brain. This causes dizziness because we rely on these senses for balance. Many people find that they get relief from dizziness by taking regular doses of apple cider vinegar tonic.

EARACHES - Earaches are normally the result of ear infections and always require the attention of a physician as soon as possible. Often there is a wait before you can get the patient to see the physician or for the effects of the medicine to take hold.

Relief from discomfort and healing benefits can be obtained by holding the affected ear over a steam bath with 1 part apple cider to two parts water. Be careful not to hold the ear too close to the steam. This is especially suited to young children who get frequent ear infections.

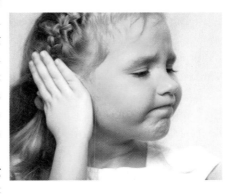

ECZEMA - Apple cider vinegar can be effective by relieving the dryness and itching of eczema. The ideal mixture is to mix it with equal parts water and apply with a dipped cotton ball.

EXHAUSTION - Exhaustion in and of itself is not considered a serious medical condition. In the short-term before recovery, it can cause a temporary but debilitating effect on your ability to perform simple tasks, and also your wellbeing. To lessen the effects and promote a speedy recovery, try a refreshing apple cider vinegar sponge bath. Run a warm bath and add as much apple cider vinegar as you can, sponge yourself regularly with the warm water, staying in the bath for at least half an hour.

FATIGUE - Apple cider vinegar is a good source of amino acids. Amino acids can help neutralize the lactic acid that builds up in our muscles and blood stream after exercise or periods of high stress. The amino acids and enzymes we get from taking regular doses of apple cider vinegar is thought to be effective in combating fatigue.

FEVER - Vinegar compresses applied to the lower legs have been recommended by physicians for many years as a means of reducing fevers. The patient is kept warm, while their lower legs are wrapped in tea towels soaked in a mixture of one part apple cider vinegar to three parts water. When the compresses dry out, they must be re-soaked and applied again. A similar folk remedy for fevers involves soaking cotton socks in the same solution and then placing them on the feet. You then wrap the patients' feet in towels to keep them warm.

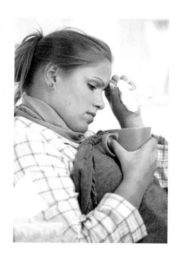

FLATULENCE - Flatulence occurs naturally in our bodies and is usually caused by swallowing air and gases produced from food that has not been digested properly. We swallow small amounts of air when we swallow our food and when we swallow our saliva. We either burp this air out through our mouths or it follows our digestive tract and is expelled from our back passage. Some foods like beans and cabbage are more likely to cause gas than others, but our individual food tolerances also play a role in what food gives us the most gas. Sipping a glass with a tablespoon of apple cider vinegar mixed with water before meals is known to aid digestion and reduce the volume and frequency of flatulence.

FOOD POISONING - Apple cider vinegar has known antibacterial properties that makes it an effective remedy for fighting off the harmful bacteria that cause food poisoning. The best method of doing this is to mix two glasses of apple cider vinegar tonic (one tablespoon apple cider vinegar per glass of water) and take small sips to finish them over an eight-hour period. In addition to this you should only drink clear fluids like tea, club soda, or water—nothing with any sugar in it like fruit juices, etc. Apple cider vinegar tonic can also be used as a preventative when visiting foreign countries, or even when going to a picnic where you are unsure of the cooking and hygiene.

FOOT CARE - We all have those hard days where we have been on our feet longer than usual and they end up swollen and sore. One of the best things to do is have a refreshing foot bath. You will need to add several cups of apple cider vinegar to a basin with warm water in it. Soak your feet for fifteen to twenty minutes. Remove your feet and let them dry in the air to maximize the cooling effect. For any other foot problems, see also *Athlete's foot* or *Corns*.

FUNGUS INFECTIONS (see also *diaper rash*) - You should use a solution of half apple cider vinegar to half water and apply several times a day until the infection is gone. A solution of half apple cider vinegar to half cooled rooibos/red bush tea is also very effective.

GALLBLADDER/GALLSTONES - Apple cider vinegar is sometimes used as part of a well-known alternative treatment, the gallbladder flush. There are a wide variety of methods and recipes for doing this but there are general similarities to all of them. Basically whole apples, apple juice, apple sauce, and apple cider vinegar tonic are the only foods or drinks ingested over a two to three day period. Once the three days is completed you then drink pure olive oil, or especially in the case of a routine flush of small stones, a mixture of olive oil and freshly squeezed and pulped grapefruit. Sometimes an enema is prescribed for the morning after the ingestion of the olive oil if the patient has not had a satisfactory bowel movement that has flushed the small gallstones. Painful gallstones should always be treated by a physician; an annual gallbladder flush generally helps avoid the formation of larger stones. The efficacy of this method of treatment is substantiated by the relative low incidence of gallbladder problems in people who consume regular amounts of apple cider vinegar tonic.

GUMS - Apple cider vinegar can be used effectively as a mouth rinse for the treatment of bleeding gums. The acidic nature of apple cider vinegar dissolves the plaque that can aggravate gums and helps fight oral infections in much the same way that it helps with cuts and scrapes.

HEADACHES - Research into headaches, especially migraines, suggests that they are caused by food we ingest or environmental stress. The food causality is triggered by eating meals made up of pizza, burgers, French fries, soft drinks, fried chicken, donuts, potato chips, pretzels, candy, etc., as these foods leave an acidic ash when digested and cause the body's pH to become acidic. Environmental stress causes stress hormones to be released into our bodies; this can lead to a condition known as acidosis. These conditions are basically when our body's pH reaches a dangerous toxic level of acidity. Supplementing your diet with apple cider vinegar tonic is known to reduce the body's acidity because when it is digested it leaves an alkaline ash, which in turn neutralizes the excess acid in our systems.

HEAD LICE - If over-the-counter lice preparations are not available or are too toxic for your skin, try rinsing your hair with full strength apple cider, then allow it to dry naturally. This will kill the adult lice and dissolve the glue that binds the eggs to the hair shaft. Now wash your hair with shampoo and then apply olive oil to your hair. The olive oil will allow you to see any remaining lice or eggs; you must then pick them out with a comb and re-wash your hair. Repeat this daily until all the lice are gone.

HEARTBURN - *See Indigestion*

HEMORRHOIDS - Apple cider vinegar can be applied in its full-strength form to hemorrhoids to reduce stinging and promote shrinking. The daily use of apple cider vinegar tonic can help to soften stools and reduce the strain during bowel movements. This will eliminate the main cause of hemorrhoids occurring.

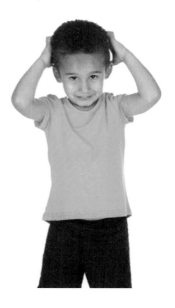

HERPES - *See Cold Sores*

HICCUPS - There are countless remedies for the treatment of hiccups, so it is of little surprise that proponents of apple cider vinegar have a few of their own. One remedy is to sip a glass of warm apple cider vinegar tonic from the far side of the glass. Another is to take a tablespoon of apple cider vinegar and mix it with a tablespoon of refined sugar and then consume. Probably one of the only instances where refined sugar is used as a remedy!

HIVES AND RASHES - You can mix apple cider vinegar with corn starch to make a paste that can be applied to rashes and hives. You can add cooled rooibos/red bush tea if available. This mixture will alleviate some of the itching and swelling.

HOARSENESS - See *sore throat.*

IMPETIGO (staph/strep infections) - Impetigo is an especially troublesome and contagious infection of the skin. It results from either a staphylococcus or streptococcus bacterial infection and is especially prevalent in young children, as they want to touch everything. To treat it with apple cider vinegar, apply it full strength to the affected skin every three hours. You should see results in a few days. If the infection persists or worsens, or there is a risk of widespread contagion, you should consult a physician as soon as possible.

INDIGESTION/HEARTBURN - Indigestion and heartburn result just as often from having too little hydrochloric acid in the stomach as having too much. It is also the movement of acid into the esophagus. Regular use of apple cider vinegar tonic will help break down proteins and fats in the stomach. It is especially useful if taken prior to a large, rich meal. This is because it stimulates saliva production which aids in the digestion of food. You should try using this remedy in place of antacid medicines, as over time these medicines will reduce the production of the necessary acids. This in turn could potentially exacerbate digestion problems and symptoms.

INSECT BITES AND STINGS - Be sure to get appropriate treatment for spider bites and other bites and stings if you are allergic. Full-strength apple cider vinegar can be used to lessen the pain and swelling of bee stings, fire ant bites, mosquito bites, wasp stings, and spider bites. You can also use it on jellyfish stings if hot water is not available or the sting is not too severe. Apple cider vinegar would definitely be a prudent addition to your luggage when visiting the beach or nature parks.

INSOMNIA - Apple cider vinegar can be used as a natural treatment for insomnia. Try making a mixture of apple cider vinegar and honey mixed with a glass of water. Keep a second glass ready for if you wake during the night. Both apple cider vinegar and honey are known to activate serotonin production in the brain which promotes relaxation and induces sleepiness.

JELLYFISH STINGS - See *Insect Bites*

JOCK ITCH - Jock itch can be treated similarly to other rashes by applying a mixture of half water to half apple cider vinegar directly to the affected area. Do this twice daily after bathing.

KIDNEY STONES - There are a few apple cider vinegar–based regimens for treating kidney stones. The common point for all of them is that you can use it in conjunction with lemon juice, but it is not essential. At the first onset of pain or discomfort, take a mixture of 2 tablespoons apple cider vinegar and 2 tablespoons of lemon juice in a glass of water. Then mix the same amount of apple cider vinegar and lemon into a 2-liter bottle of water. Drink a glass of this mixture every hour until the stone has passed. Refill the bottle with the mixture as often as necessary and keep drinking. If you feel the stone is stuck, you can add two tablespoons of olive oil to the glass.

LAMENESS - Dr. Jarvis had a favorite remedy for sore, tired legs. One tablespoon apple cider vinegar combined with the yolk of one egg and one tablespoon of turpentine. To be applied daily to the legs as needed.

LARYNGITIS - *See Sore Throat*

LEG CRAMPS - Leg cramps are usually a sign of an electrolyte imbalance such as a deficiency in magnesium and calcium, or a deficiency in vitamin E. Taking a regular daily tonic of apple cider vinegar will supply your body with some of the minerals and vitamins it lacks.

LIVER FUNCTION - The liver is one of the most important organs in the body as it filters out toxins and waste products from the blood. To improve liver function you can cleanse the liver with an apple cider vinegar detox. This is in addition to taking the daily apple cider tonic. The night before you begin your detox day, have a light, easy-to-digest dinner of steamed vegetables and fish. The following morning you only ingest liquids such as vegetable juices, broths, apple juice, green tea, and other healthy liquids. Up the daily tonic to morning and evening, or if you already take it that way, double the dosage. The week following your detox day, eat only fresh foods with no preservatives added.

LONGEVITY - Visible signs of aging are just as likely to be caused by a poor metabolism and acidic body pH as it is from chronological age. Studies in aging are beginning to link an acidic body pH to cell degeneration and the bodies' poor response to free radicals. Taking a daily tonic can help restore your pH to healthier levels and improve your metabolism.

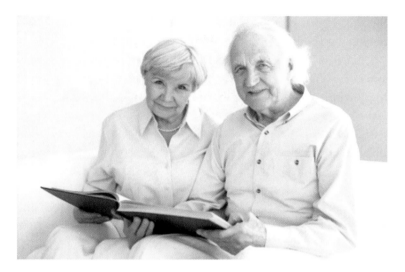

MEMORY - Apple cider vinegar is known to help the body metabolize iron and provides trace amounts of amino acids. Iron helps carry oxygen to the cells and amino acids are essential in the synthesis of brain chemicals. Both of these factors are known to aid memory function. The feeling among experts is that people who take a regular dose of apple cider vinegar tonic have consistently good mental powers even as they age.

MENSTRUAL PROBLEMS - The regular daily tonic of apple cider vinegar can help lessen the flow of a heavy period. It can in some cases make your period late, so it is advised to stop taking it up to three or four days prior to when it is expected.

MORNING SICKNESS - Like indigestion is at times a problem of too little stomach acid, morning sickness is sometimes the result of too little stomach acid. This is caused by there being no stimulus to produce digestive acids after a night of inactivity.

Sipping a glass of apple cider vinegar tonic in the morning can help bring about a comfortable balance of stomach acids.

MUSCLE SORENESS AND STIFF JOINTS - You can apply apple cider vinegar directly to stiff muscles and sore joints to alleviate pain. It is also effective when added to your bath if you soak in it for thirty minutes. You can also soak compresses with it. Taking the daily tonic will also help with any electrolyte imbalance that may be contributing to the discomfort.

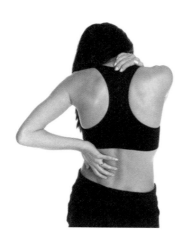

NASAL CONGESTION - *See Colds*

NAUSEA - *See Morning Sickness*

NETTLES - *See Poison Ivy*

NERVOUS TIC - Regular doses of apple cider vinegar can help provide the minerals that regulate our nervous systems.

NEURALGIA - Regular doses of apple cider vinegar can help balance the body's pH and therefore help the immune system's response to this condition.

NIGHT SWEATS - For night sweats that are a result of a waning cold or the flu, try having an apple cider sponge bath before going to bed. This can also be helpful to menopausal women whose night sweats are caused by the normal rebalancing of hormones at this time of their lives. Drinking the usual glass of apple cider vinegar tonic in the morning can help to regulate the toxins that are being eliminated from your body.

NOSEBLEEDS - *See Bleeding.*

POISON IVY AND POISON OAK (see also *nettles*) - As with most other rashes, itches, and insect bites, apple cider vinegar is known to be an effective treatment. It can be used in a half water, half apple cider vinegar mixture which you dab on directly with a soaked cotton ball. Another remedy is to mix it half and half with freshly brewed and cooled rooibos/red bush tea, which in itself is an effective rash remedy. This mixture is also applied directly with a soaked cotton ball. Patricia Bragg recommended keeping a spray bottle of apple cider vinegar mix in the refrigerator as the cool temperature of the spray will add extra relief.

PYELITIS (inflammation of the kidneys) - A kidney infection is a serious medical condition and should be treated by a physician. The apple cider vinegar tonic is good to take as a preventative for kidney problems and also as a supplement to what your physician prescribes for you. Dr. Jarvis claimed to have good results treating pyelitis using the daily apple cider vinegar tonic.

RASHES- *See Hives, Poison Ivy, and Diaper Rashes.*

SHINGLES - Shingles is a painful condition that affects the nerves of the skin. Dr. Jarvis advised applying full-strength apple cider vinegar directly onto the affected areas six to eight times over a twenty-four hour period, even through the night. This treatment will probably cause a little itching and burning, which will pass quickly while promoting healing.

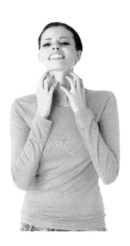

SINUSITIS - *See Colds and Flu*

SORE THROAT (also laryngitis) - Apple cider vinegar remedies for sore throats range from mixing the usual one tablespoon with a glass of water to using equal parts water to vinegar. In both cases the mixture is to be gargled and not swallowed. This is to prevent you from swallowing the germs that are causing the infection. Use these gargles or rinses hourly until symptoms subside. This is good for treating and preventing sore throats, if you know that you are going to be putting a lot of stress on your throat. It can also reduce the flow of mucus and minimize swelling.

SUNBURN AND WINDBURN - *See Burns*

SWIMMER'S EAR - You can combine the drying effect of alcohol with the disinfectant qualities of apple cider vinegar. Using three to four drops in each ear after swimming or showering will reduce the itching and pain of swimmers ear.

THRUSH - *See Fungus*

TINNITUS - Tinnitus is a condition that results in a constant ringing in the ears; the cause of the condition is not fully understood. A daily dose of the apple cider vinegar tonic is thought to help by improving circulation and the mineral balance in our bodies.

TOOTH DECAY (see also *gums and bleeding*) - Rinsing daily with a glass of apple cider vinegar tonic can help maintain good oral hygiene and fight the bacteria that lead to tooth decay and gum disease.

ULCERS - Preliminary studies have indicated that ingesting a weak concentration of apple cider vinegar can help stimulate the digestive system to combat ulcers.

URINARY PROBLEMS (see also *bladder*) - Drinking the apple cider vinegar tonic before every meal can help regulate urine production and protect the kidneys from infection.

VARICOSE VEINS - Many apple cider vinegar experts espouse the use of compresses soaked in apple cider vinegar to treat varicose veins. You wrap the legs twice a day and keep them elevated for half an hour. This is in conjunction with the tonic with every meal.

WARTS - Make a mixture of one part salt to four parts apple cider and apply it several times a day to the warts until they disappear.

YEAST INFECTIONS - Use a douche of 2 tablespoons apple cider vinegar to 1 quart warm water, twice daily until the symptoms have stopped. Adding a cup of apple cider vinegar to your bath will provide external relief.

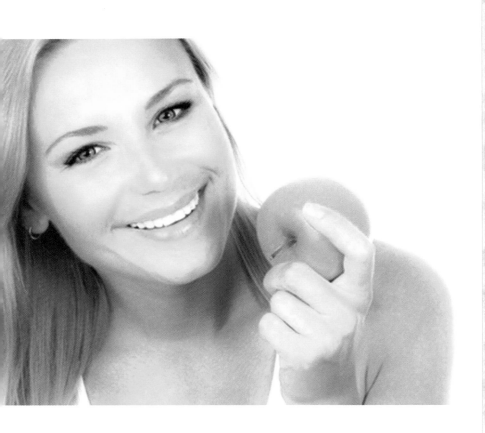

Apple Cider Vinegar and A Beautiful You

Apple cider vinegar's effectiveness as a weight loss accelerator and as a remedy for many ailments is well established. However it is a lesser known fact that it is also an effective cosmetic aid. The surface of our skin is naturally slightly acidic, but most of the soaps we use leave it in an alkaline state. This is obviously not desirable as it opens the door for many bacteria and other ailments. Apple cider vinegar can help your skin regain its protective qualities and leave it looking beautiful and radiant.

You too can have the beautiful glow of a polished apple without resorting to expensive chemicals and commercial cosmetics. Use it in your bath or shower, use it on your face or any area of your body that is under attack from bacteria or fungus. Use it to remove unwanted oils from your body and nails. Apple cider vinegar has a proven track record in detoxifying and benefitting the skin by removing unwanted substances and helping return your skin to its correct pH.

Remember beauty comes from within and a healthy, balanced system that is regularly cleansed and fortified with apple cider vinegar will leave you feeling healthy and energetic. This can only have a positive effect on all aspects of your life.

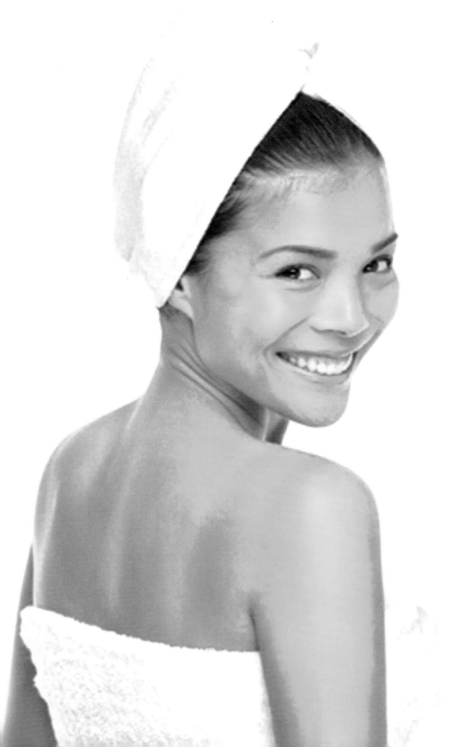

In the Bath

One of the most common ways to use apple cider vinegar is when you bathe or shower. This is because it helps regulate the natural pH of our skin. There are many different recipes for hot apple cider vinegar detoxification and skin conditioning baths, but one of the more common and most effective recipes is to combine 1 cup of apple cider vinegar with 1 tablespoon of ginger. Another is 1 cup of apple cider vinegar combined with 3 cups of kosher salt. Add these to a bath of water as hot as you can comfortably stand and soak for thirty minutes and then rinse yourself off. You can also keep a plastic bottle of apple cider vinegar inside your shower stall so you can apply it to your skin either with a wash cloth or a cupped hand. The clean refreshing tingle you feel afterwards will probably surprise you!

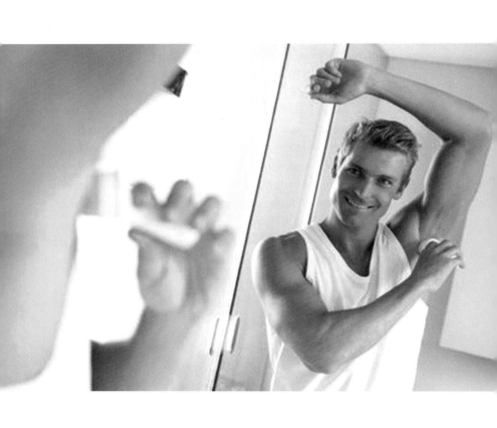

Healthy Deodorant

Apple cider vinegar can also be used in the place of deodorizing soap. This is because it provides an acidic barrier on your skin that fights bacteria and other odor-causing germs. This can reduce our reliance on deodorants that can irritate the skin and will also leave your skin with a clean fresh scent. Simply splash some apple cider vinegar onto your underarms and wait for it to dry, or, using an old roll-on bottle, wash, fill with apple cider vinegar and roll under your arms. The strong fragrance of the apple cider vinegar will fade completely as it dries.

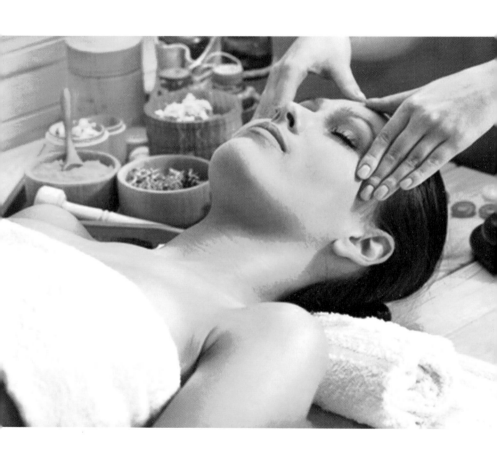

Facial Care

Apple cider vinegar can also be part of your regular facial as it can be useful in removing dead skin cells and can help to prevent acne and other skin blemishes. You can make a steam facial by adding ½ cup of apple cider vinegar to a bowl of very hot water, then covering your head with a towel and bending over the bowl. Now use a wash cloth or a cleansing pad to wipe away the oil and dirt. Remember to splash your face with cold water afterwards to close your pores.

Another method for cleansing your pores is by rinsing a hand towel in hot water and then covering your face with it for a few minutes. Now remove the hand towel and cover your face with a tea towel soaked in warm water with a few tablespoons of apple cider vinegar added. After this, cover the tea towel with a freshly soaked and warmed hand towel. Rub your face clean as you remove the combination of towels. Once again use a wash cloth or a cleansing pad to wipe away the oil and dirt, remembering to splash your face with cold water afterwards to close your pores.

You can also make a pretty awesome face mask by combining equal parts apple cider vinegar with Aztec Secret Indian Healing Clay. Leave this detoxifying, deep-pore treatment on for ten to fifteen minutes before rinsing it off with warm water.

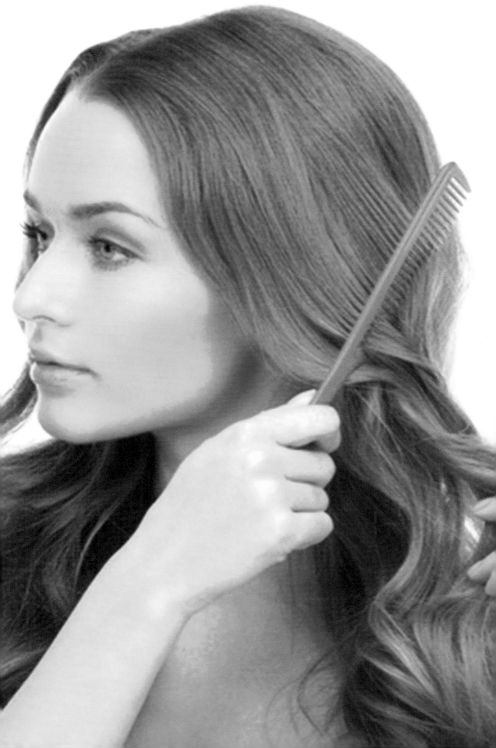

Hair Care

An effective use for apple cider vinegar is for treating lice infestations. You pour apple cider vinegar onto dry hair, making sure to coat the hair thoroughly, and then leave it to dry naturally. This dissolves the glue that causes the lice eggs to cling to the hair shaft. After this you need to spread olive oil through the hair, then remove as many of the dead lice and eggs as possible by hand. Wash and rinse the hair with shampoo and conditioner to remove any you may have missed.

You can also use the classic application for apple cider vinegar as a natural rinse. I recommend recycling an old shampoo bottle and adding 1 tablespoon of apple cider vinegar to 2 cups of cold water for restoring the shine and luster to tired, damaged hair and for loosening tangles. Apple cider vinegar is also effective in controlling the bacteria that causes dandruff; just add ¼ cup to 1 quart of warm water and use it as a final rinse.

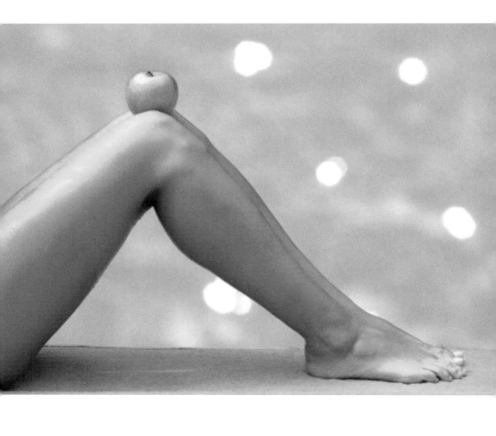

Feet and Legs

Apple cider vinegar can be used effectively to make you more beautiful from head to toe—literally—so best not neglect your feet! It can be used to treat calluses and corns, as well as reduce foot odor and invigorate tired feet. To make a refreshing foot soak, add a ¼ to a ½ cup of apple cider vinegar to a basin of lukewarm water and soak your feet daily for about ten minutes. The acidity of the apple cider vinegar will also help destroy the bacteria that causes foot odor and the fungus that leads to athlete's foot. To treat corns and calluses, the concentration of vinegar needs to be higher and you need to soak for at least half an hour. Once your feet are dry from the soak, you can use a pumice stone to rub away the corns and calluses. Pumice stones are available from most health shops.

For those who use nail polish, try rubbing your nails clean with a cotton ball dipped in apple cider vinegar before applying the nail polish. The vinegar will dissolve and remove any residual oils on your nails and thus help the polish last longer. The apple cider vinegar will also promote healthy cuticles and nails.

It is an unfortunate fact of life that most of us will develop varicose veins in our legs as we get older. Try this old folk remedy before you go for any of the expensive modern remedies on the market. Soak some tea towels in apple cider vinegar and then wrap them around your legs. Now elevate your legs for half an hour, leaving the wrappings on.

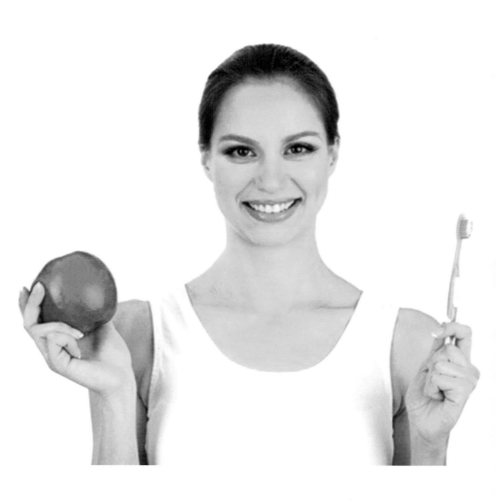

Oral Health

To freshen your breath and cleanse your mouth of bacteria, try swishing and gargling with the following mixture: A ¼ cup of coconut oil, melted and then cooled, 1 tablespoon of apple cider vinegar, and 1 tablespoon of lemon juice. Do this for a minimum of three minutes, using up all the mixture as you go. This is best done at night, before going to bed.

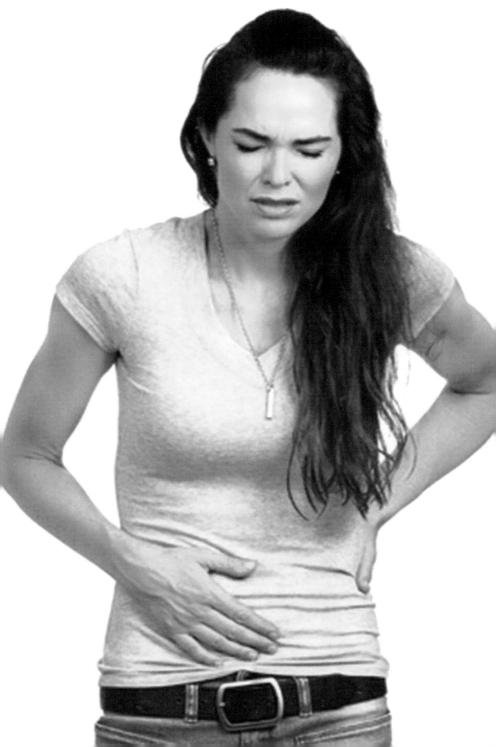

Side Effects of Apple Cider Vinegar

Apple cider vinegar is a powerful substance, which is precisely why it is such an effective remedy for so many ailments. However, with power comes responsibility. Even when used correctly as prescribed, there can be side effects from the reactions that apple cider vinegar precipitates in your body. When detoxing the liver using the liver cleanse described in the Common Ailments section above, you could expect to have headaches, nausea, and lightheadedness. These conditions are caused by the toxins leaving the body and are actually a positive sign, meaning the detox/cleanse is working. When using full-strength apple cider vinegar as a remedy on your skin, you can experience a burning sensation; this is indicative of how strong apple cider vinegar is and of its effectiveness. Caution should be exercised to ensure you don't use too much for too long in any remedy as this may harm you. Taking full-strength apple cider vinegar on a regular basis can be harmful to your teeth by dissolving the calcium in them. Apple cider vinegar should always be used as instructed as improper use can lead to damaging side effects.

When dealing with serious infections, injury, chronic ailments, or diseases, you should always consult a physician as a first course of action. You should then discuss supplementing whatever treatment they prescribe with an apple cider vinegar tonic or remedy. Apple cider vinegar is of course also an effective bridging treatment until medical help is available.

Apple cider vinegar is a powerful and effective medicinal agent when used correctly. Even so the user must be vigilant for side effects, as each person's body is different and responds in its own unique way to everything it comes into contact with. This applies even more so when apple cider is not used as indicated for any particular ailment. As with anything, common sense must prevail—if you feel something is not right or you are experiencing side effects that are out of the ordinary, discontinue use and consult your doctor. Having said this, experiencing side effects with apple cider vinegar is a rarity and certainly not the norm. The vast majority of people can take apple cider vinegar regularly without any kind of adverse reaction.

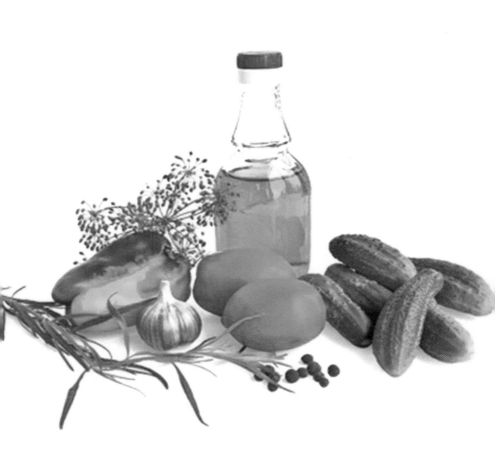

Cooking with Apple Cider Vinegar

Apple cider vinegar has many uses, but one of the easiest ways to up your daily intake is to use it in your cooking. It adds a new dimension to otherwise bland recipes, and is so versatile it can be included in everything from salads to condiments to main meals and even in desserts and drinks. I have compiled an amazing selection of recipes to whet your appetite and get you started in the kitchen as you embark on your apple cider vinegar journey. I hope you enjoy these as much as I did.

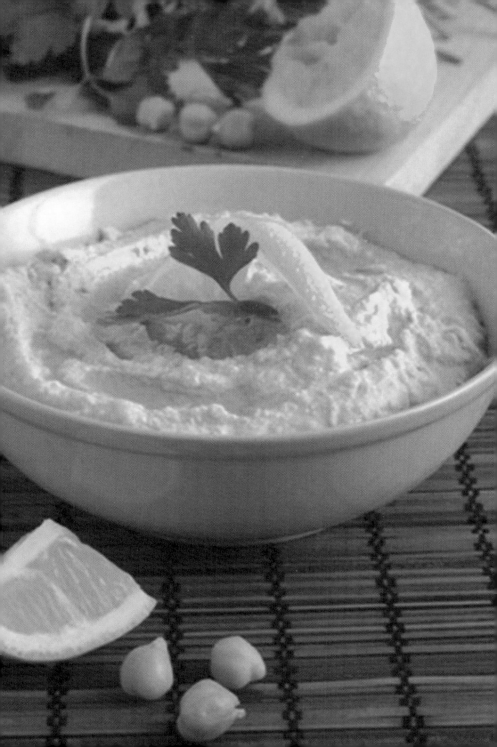

Dips

Quick Hummus

Yields: 1½ cups

Ingredients:

15 ounces canned chickpeas, drained and rinsed

¼ cup olive oil

3 garlic cloves

3 tablespoons lemon juice, freshly squeezed

2 tablespoons tahini

1–2 tablespoons water

1 tablespoon organic apple cider vinegar

2 teaspoons cumin

½ teaspoon paprika

Salt to taste

Directions:

1. Place the chickpeas, olive oil, garlic cloves, lemon juice, tahini, apple cider vinegar, cumin, and salt into the food processor and blend until smooth and creamy adding a few drops of water at a time until the desired consistency is reached.
2. Transfer to a bowl, sprinkle with the paprika and serve with your choice of dippers.
3. YUM!

Walnut Paté

Walnuts are a great source of Omega-3s, protein, and antioxidants.

Yields: 1 cup

Ingredients:

1 cup walnuts, soaked in water
  overnight, then drained
¼ cup organic apple, peeled
  and chopped
2 tablespoons cilantro,
  chopped

1 garlic clove
1 teaspoon lemon juice
1 teaspoon organic apple cider
  vinegar
¼ teaspoon sea salt

Directions:

1. Combine all the ingredients in a food processor and process until smooth and creamy.
2. Serve this delicious paté on a bed of organic greens, as a dip for fresh veggie sticks, or as a sandwich filling on dehydrated bread.

Cashew Cheese Dip

Yields: 1 cup

Ingredients:

¾ cup cashews, soaked in
    water overnight and then
    drained
¼ cup water
2 tablespoons lemon juice
½ teaspoon organic apple cider
    vinegar

1 teaspoon nutritional yeast
1 garlic clove
¼ teaspoon sea salt
Pinch of ground black pepper

Directions:

1. Add all the ingredients to a food processor and blend until smooth and creamy.
2. This dip is absolutely delicious served with fresh veggie crudités.

Roasted Red Pepper and Onion Dip

Yields: 1½ cups

Ingredients:

8 ounces low fat cream cheese, softened

3 red peppers, cut into strips

1 large onion, cut into eighths

2 tablespoons olive oil

2 tablespoons organic apple cider vinegar

½ teaspoon garlic powder

½ teaspoon onion powder

Salt and pepper to taste

Directions:

1. Preheat the oven to 450°F.
2. Place the onions and red pepper strips into a bowl and toss them together with the olive oil, apple cider vinegar, garlic powder, onion powder, salt, and pepper.
3. Place the whole mixture into an oven-proof dish and bake for 20 minutes or until the peppers are fork-tender.
4. Remove from the oven and allow to cool down.
5. Throw the veggie mixture into the blender with the cream cheese and purée until smooth.
6. Add more salt and pepper if needed, then cover and refrigerate until needed.
7. Allow the dip to come to room temperature and soften before serving with assorted veggies and/or chips for dipping.
8. Enjoy!

Smoked Salmon and Horseradish Dip

Yields: about 1 cup

Ingredients:

¼ pound smoked salmon, chopped

8 ounces low fat cream cheese, softened

2 tablespoons horseradish

2 tablespoons fresh dill, chopped

2 tablespoons lemon juice, freshly squeezed

1 teaspoon organic apple cider vinegar

Salt and pepper to taste

Directions:

1. Stir the horseradish, dill, lemon juice, apple cider vinegar, salt, and pepper into the cream cheese vigorously.
2. When thoroughly combined, fold in the salmon gently.
3. Serve with your choice of dippers.
4. Enjoy!

Broccoli and Bacon Dip

Yields: about 2½ cups

Ingredients:

4 pieces bacon

14 ounces broccoli, cut into florets

1 cup low fat cream cheese, softened

1 teaspoon garlic powder

½ teaspoon organic apple cider vinegar

Directions:

1. Fry the bacon in a nonstick skillet until it is crispy. Set it aside on paper towels to drain and cool. Once cool enough to handle, crumble it into small pieces.
2. Steam the broccoli florets until they are tender, but not mushy.
3. Put the broccoli and the cream cheese into the food processor along with the garlic powder and apple cider vinegar and purée until smooth.
4. Transfer to your serving bowl and sprinkle the crumbled bacon over the top.
5. Serve with your chips of choice.
6. Superb!

Flavors of the Orient Dip

Yields: about 1½ cups

Ingredients:

½ cup fresh ginger, grated
½ cup olive oil
2 bunches of cilantro, thick
    stems removed
3 tablespoons organic apple
    cider vinegar

3 tablespoons soy sauce
    (preferably low sodium, or
    substitute coconut aminos)
2 teaspoons sesame oil

Directions:

1. Place all the ingredients into the food processor and blend until smooth.
2. This is a fantastic dip to accompany shrimp.
3. Finger-licking good!

Dill and Horseradish Dip

Yields: about 1½ cups

Ingredients:

8 ounces low fat cream cheese, softened

¼ cup prepared horseradish

3 tablespoons fresh dill, chopped

2 tablespoons low fat milk

1 tablespoon organic apple cider vinegar

Salt to taste

Directions:

1. In a bowl, beat the horseradish, cream cheese, apple cider vinegar, milk, and salt until light and fluffy, then gently fold in the dill.
2. Serve with your choice of dippers.
3. Enjoy!

Caramelized Onion and Thyme Dip

Yields: about 2 cups

Ingredients:

2 onions, sliced thinly
2 tablespoons organic butter
1 cup sour cream
⅛ cup organic apple cider
    vinegar

8 ounces low fat cream cheese,
    softened
2 tablespoons fresh thyme,
    chopped
Salt and pepper to taste

Directions:

1. Melt the butter in a nonstick skillet, then add the onions, salt, and pepper and cook over a medium-low heat for 30 minutes, stirring occasionally until they are golden brown.
2. Remove the onions from the pan and set aside to cool.
3. Turn the heat up and add the apple cider vinegar to deglaze the pan, taking care to scrape up all the browned bits off the bottom. Allow the liquid to reduce by half then pour it into a bowl and allow it to cool.
4. Once cool, mix the onions, the deglazing liquid, the cream cheese, and the thyme together in a bowl.
5. Add more salt and pepper if desired and serve with your choice of dippers.

Note: If you don't like a chunky dip, throw it all into the blender and purée until smooth before serving.

Good Old Fashioned Guacamole with a Twist

Yields: 2 cups

Ingredients:

2 avocados, diced

½ red onion, finely chopped

¼ cup fresh cilantro, chopped

2 tablespoons organic apple
    cider vinegar

2 tablespoons lime juice,
    freshly squeezed

1 teaspoon red pepper flakes,
    or to taste

Salt and black pepper to taste

Directions:

1. Mix all the ingredients together in a bowl. Leave the avocado pieces in cubes for a chunkier guacamole, or mash it up with a fork if you prefer.
2. Serve immediately with your favorite dippers.
3. Amazing!

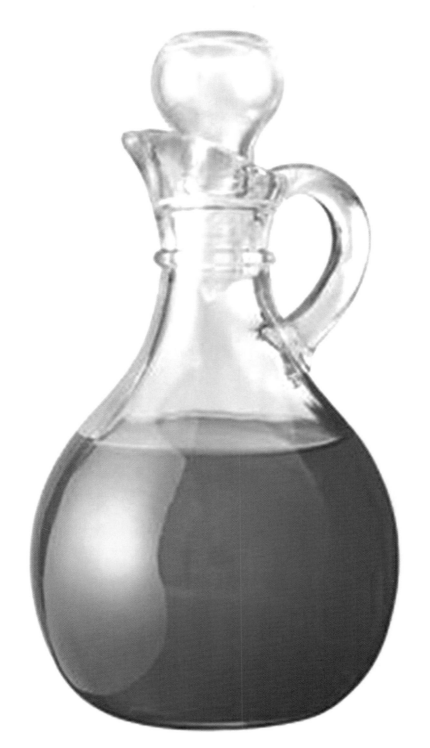

Salad Dressings and Condiments

Homemade Salad Dressing

I like the clean flavor of olive oil with apple cider vinegar. The sweetener will help you soften the "bite" of this amount of vinegar, if you prefer.

Yields: ³⁄₄ cup

Ingredients:

½ cup olive oil

⅓ cup organic apple cider vinegar

¼ teaspoon salt

1 teaspoon raw organic honey or maple syrup (optional)

1 garlic clove, crushed

½ teaspoon dry mustard

½ teaspoon paprika

¼ teaspoon black pepper

Directions:

1. Combine all the ingredients in a jar, shake, and serve. *Do not refrigerate.*

Sweet and Sour Sauce

Yields: about 3 cups

Ingredients:

¼ cup organic apple cider
    vinegar
¾ cup vegetable broth
1 tablespoon tomato paste
1 tablespoon soy sauce
1 tablespoon molasses or maple
    syrup

¼ cup Sucanat
1 (7-ounce) can crushed
    pineapple
1 tablespoon cornstarch
¼ cup water

Directions:

1. Mix all the ingredients in a medium saucepan.
2. Bring to a boil and then simmer until thickened.
3. Store in the fridge until needed.

Barbecue Sauce

Yields: 3 quarts

Ingredients:

4 cups vegetable stock
3 (14-ounce) bottles chili sauce
1 teaspoon cayenne pepper
1 teaspoon dry mustard
1½ cups organic apple cider
   vinegar

1 garlic clove
4 teaspoons salt
6 tablespoons lemon juice
2 cups olive oil
½ cup organic plain flour
½ cup cold water

Directions:

1. Combine all the ingredients, except the flour and cold water, in a large saucepan and cook slowly for about 30 minutes.
2. Whisk together the flour and cold water, then stir the mixture into the sauce to thicken it.
3. Store in bottles in the fridge until needed.

Zesty Mustard

If you've never made your own mustard before, try this simple recipe. You can experiment with adding chopped fresh herbs and crushed garlic for a different flavor dimension if you like.

Yields: about 3 cups

Ingredients:

1 cup organic apple cider
    vinegar
1 cup dry mustard

2 eggs, beaten
½ cup rapadura
Pinch of salt

Directions:

1. Combine the apple cider vinegar and mustard in a glass bowl, then cover and let stand overnight.
2. Pour the mixture into a medium saucepan and stir in the remaining ingredients.
3. Bring to a slow boil, stirring constantly.
4. Cook until thick, then cool and refrigerate.
5. Keeps for about 4 weeks.

Note: Try adding some whole mustard seeds for a different texture.

Red Pepper Jam

Yields: about 14 half-pints

Ingredients:

12 large red bell peppers
1 tablespoon sea salt
3 cups rapadura

2 cups organic apple cider
vinegar

Directions:

1. Wash the peppers, remove the seeds, and cut them into quarters.
2. Add the red peppers to the food processor and mince finely.
3. Sprinkle with the salt and allow to stand for 4 hours.
4. Drain the pepper mixture and add the rapadura and apple cider vinegar.
5. Cook over a medium heat until thick, about 1 hour.
6. Pour into hot, sterilized half-pint jars, and seal with sterilized canning lids.
7. Use as desired.

Dill Pickles

Yields: 1 quart

Ingredients:

1 quart of cucumbers, approximately 3–4 inches in length

1 teaspoon mustard seeds

1 cup organic apple cider vinegar

2 cups water

1 tablespoon coarse sea salt

1 teaspoon dill seed, or 3 heads fresh dill

Directions:

1. Scrub the cucumbers well and pack into hot, sterilized canning jars.
2. Add either the dill seed or heads of fresh dill.
3. Combine the rest of the ingredients in a saucepan to make the brine and bring to a boil over a medium high heat.
4. Immediately ladle the brine over the cucumbers, filling the jars to within ½ an inch of the top of the rim.
5. Top with sterilized caps and rings, and seal tightly.
6. Cool away from drafts.
7. Serve as desired.

Pickled Apples

These make a delicious accompaniment to winter meals.

Yields: 7 pints

Ingredients:

4 cups organic apple cider vinegar

2 cups water

6 cups rapadura

2 tablespoons whole cloves

4 cinnamon sticks, broken into bits

8 pounds small apples, cored and peeled

Directions:

1. Combine the apple cider vinegar, water, and rapadura in a large stock pot.
2. Wrap the cloves and cinnamon sticks in cheesecloth or place them in a stainless steel tea strainer submerged in the liquid. (Do not use aluminum.)
3. Boil until the rapadura has dissolved, then add the whole apples and simmer until tender, about 30 minutes.
4. Remove the pot from the heat and let it sit for 12 to 18 hours so the flavors will meld.
5. Pack the apples into 7 sterilized pint jars.
6. Remove the spices from the syrup, then bring the syrup back to a boil.

7. Once boiling, remove from the heat and ladle into the jars to about a ¼ inch from the top.
8. Cover with canning lids and process in boiling water for 10 minutes.
9. Remove the jars and cool on a thick towel or wire rack.
10. Be sure the lids have sealed completely before storing.

Strawberry Vinaigrette

This unusual dressing is the perfect accompaniment to a kale, spinach, or arugula based salad.

Yields: about 2 cups

Ingredients:

10 ounces sugar-free straw-
    berry preserves
½ cup fresh strawberries
¼ cup water
¼ cup organic apple cider
    vinegar

¼ cup macadamia oil
    (or substitute olive oil)
3 teaspoons honey
2 teaspoons chia seeds

Directions:

1. Place all the ingredients into the blender and purèe to your desired consistency by adding more or less water.
2. Refrigerate before using.
3. Use within 3 days.

Simple Apple Cider Vinaigrette

This simple vinaigrette is incredibly versatile. Not just content to liven up salad greens, you can use this as a sauce for seafood, green vegetables, and poultry.

Yields: about 2 cups

Ingredients:

1 cup organic apple cider vinegar

1 cup olive oil

½ cup freshly squeezed lemon juice

½ cup cilantro, roughly chopped

4 tablespoons Dijon mustard

1 tablespoon mild curry powder (optional)

1 garlic clove, peeled

Directions:

1. Place the apple cider vinegar, lemon juice, cilantro, Dijon mustard, curry powder, and garlic clove into your food processor and blend until well combined.
2. Now slowly, with the blender still running, pour in the olive oil and pulse continuously until the dressing has emulsified.
3. Store in the fridge and use as needed.
4. Keeps for 4–5 days.

Holiday Jam

Try this gently spiced festive cranberry jam all year round.

Yields: 5 pints

Ingredients:

12 cups fresh cranberries

3 cups organic apple cider
vinegar

2 cups organic granulated
sugar (or sugar substitute)

Juice of 1 lemon

Zest of 1 lemon

Juice of 2 oranges

Zest of 1 orange

2 tablespoons cinnamon

1 tablespoon grated ginger

1 teaspoon nutmeg

½ teaspoon ground cloves

Directions:

1. Combine the cranberries and all the other liquid ingredients and zest in a pot. Make sure it is a fairly big one as this jam can bubble over when heated.
2. Bring the pot to the boil and remove any foam that settles on the top from the fruit.
3. Cook for about 15 minutes or until the cranberries pop, then add the spices and mix in well.
4. Cook until the jam is quite thick, stirring often.
5. Spoon the jam into sterilized jam jars and seal them, then process them in a boiling water bath for 10 minutes.
6. Store in a cool place and use within a week once opened.

Sage and Caramelized Onion Relish

Yields: 1 Serving

Ingredients:

2 onions, chopped

3 tablespoons organic apple
  cider vinegar

2 tablespoons raw honey

2 tablespoons olive oil

2 tablespoons butter

2 tablespoons fresh sage,
  chopped

Salt and pepper to taste

Directions:

1. Heat up the butter and olive oil in a saucepan over a medium heat.
2. Add the onions and sauté for about 5 minutes, until they are just beginning to soften, then stir in the remaining ingredients.
3. Cover and cook over a low heat for a further 20 minutes, stirring occasionally.
4. Now remove the lid, and increase the heat to medium high. Cook, stirring often, for another 20 minutes or until the onions are golden and caramelized.
5. Season with salt and pepper and then remove from the heat and allow to cool down.
6. Serve with pork, turnips, or roast ham or simply on some healthy bread; however you prefer, it's delicious!

Classic Strawberry Jam

Yields: 1 pint

Ingredients:

3 cups fresh strawberries, chopped

1 cup sweet red wine

1 cup rapadura

2 tablespoons organic apple cider vinegar

2 tablespoons fresh ginger, grated

2 tablespoons cinnamon

Directions:

1. Place the strawberries in a bowl and pour over the red wine. Allow the strawberries to marinate for about 10 minutes, then transfer the whole mixture to a large heavy-bottomed saucepan.
2. Bring to a boil and as soon as it starts, add the remaining ingredients and give everything a good stir to combine.
3. Reduce the heat to medium and boil until the jam starts to thicken. Stir the mixture every 10 minutes to prevent it from sticking and/or burning.
4. Once the jam has thickened, remove it from the heat and decant into sterilized canning jars.
5. Store it in the fridge.

Fig Chutney

Yields: about 1½ cups

Ingredients:

1 cup dried figs, roughly
    chopped
½ cup fig preserves
½ cup balsamic vinegar
¼ cup honey
1 onion, chopped

2 tablespoons organic apple
    cider vinegar
1 tablespoon butter
1 tablespoon fresh thyme,
    chopped
Salt and pepper to taste

Directions:

1. Melt the butter in a large saucepan and sauté the onion until soft, about 5 minutes.
2. Add the figs, balsamic, apple cider vinegar, honey, salt, and pepper and bring to a boil, then reduce the heat and simmer for about 15 minutes or until most of the liquid has evaporated, stirring occasionally.
3. Remove the pan from the heat and stir in the preserves and thyme, cover and allow to cool for half an hour.
4. Best served immediately, but will hold for up to a week in an airtight container in the fridge.
5. Serve with roasted pork for a real taste sensation!

Spicy Apple Jam

This versatile jam is delicious spread onto muffins, crumpets, and toast, or as a side to a pork dish.

Yields: about 4 cups

Ingredients:

4 pounds apples, peeled, cored and chopped

2 cups organic apple cider vinegar

½ cup honey or maple syrup

3 tablespoons cinnamon

1 tablespoon nutmeg

1 tablespoon allspice

1 teaspoon ground cloves

Directions:

1. Place the apples, apple cider vinegar, and honey into a large pot and cook over a low heat until soft. This can take some time so be patient.
2. Once the apples are soft and the liquid has been absorbed, pass the apple mixture through a sieve to get rid of any clumps.
3. Place the apple pulp into a clean saucepan and stir in all the spices until well mixed.
4. Now cook the apple pulp over a medium heat until it has thickened, then decant the jam into sterilized jars.
5. Once sealed, process them in a boiling water bath for 10 minutes.
6. Enjoy as desired.

Piccalilli

Yields: about 6 cups

Ingredients:

2 pounds cauliflower, cut into florets

3 cups organic apple cider vinegar

1 ½ cups green beans, ends trimmed and cut into 1-inch lengths

½ cup rapadura

½ cup organic plain flour

¼ cup cooking salt

¼ cup water

1 red onion, roughly chopped

1 red pepper, seeds removed and roughly chopped

2 cucumbers, peeled, quartered and cut into 1-inch cubes

6 garlic cloves, minced

1 tablespoon mustard seeds

1 tablespoon mustard powder

1 tablespoon fresh ginger, grated

2 teaspoons turmeric

Directions:

1. Mix the vegetables together in a bowl and sprinkle them with ⅓ of the salt, then leave them to drain for 1 hour. Rinse, drain well, and repeat another two times.

2. Combine the apple cider vinegar, rapadura, garlic, and ginger in a saucepan and bring to a boil, stirring, until all the rapadura has dissolved.

3. Once the liquid is ready, add the veggies, cover, and bring to a boil again. Once boiling, remove the lid, reduce the heat, and simmer for a further 10 minutes.
4. Place the mustard powder, mustard seeds, flour, and water in a bowl and stir together to make a paste.
5. Add the paste to the pot of vegetables and stir it in well. Allow to cook until the mixture begins to thicken.
6. Ladle the piccalilli into sterilized canning jars and seal while it is still hot.
7. A firm favorite!

Pickled Onions

Serve these delicious tangy onions as is, or jazz up this basic recipe with your choice of flavors, spices, and herbs. Some fabulous additions include cinnamon, red pepper flakes, chili powder, garlic, mustard seeds, bay leaves, ginger, coriander, fennel, or cumin to name a few. Have fun experimenting!

Yields: 3 cups

Ingredients:

3 red onions, peeled, halved, and thinly sliced

1 cup organic apple cider vinegar

½ cup freshly squeezed lime juice

¼ cup rapadura

8 whole cloves

2 tablespoons salt

Directions:

1. Separate the onions into their individual half rings and place them into a large bowl.
2. Pour enough boiling water over them to just cover them and leave them for 20 seconds and then drain.
3. Place the onions into jars.
4. Place the cloves into a saucepan and heat over a medium heat until fragrant and then whisk in the remaining ingredients.

5. Bring the brining liquid to a gentle simmer and stir until the rapadura and salt have dissolved.
6. Pour the brine over the onions.
7. Allow the jars to stand at room temperature until they are cool, then seal and place in the fridge until needed.
8. These onions hold for 2 weeks in the fridge but I doubt that they will last that long—they are totally addictive!

Tomato Ketchup

Yields: 8 servings

Ingredients:

3 pounds tomatoes, chopped

2 red onions, chopped

4 garlic cloves—minced

2 whole cloves

1 tablespoon black peppercorns

1 tablespoon mustard seeds

1 tablespoon smoked paprika

¼ teaspoon chili powder

¼ cup organic apple cider vinegar

¼ cup rapadura

¼ cup lemon juice, freshly squeezed

Salt to taste

Directions:

1. Place the tomatoes, onions, garlic, cloves, peppercorns, mustard seeds, paprika, and chili powder into a pot and bring to a boil. Once boiling, reduce the heat and allow the mixture to simmer for about 45 minutes or until half of the liquid has evaporated.

2. Remove from the heat and allow to cool down, then place it all into the blender and puree until smooth.

3. Pass the puree through a sieve, straining as much liquid as possible from the pulp into a clean saucepan.

4. Heat up the strained liquid over a medium heat and once warm, add the apple cider vinegar, rapadura, lemon juice, and salt.

5. Stir well and allow this mixture to simmer for 15 minutes or until it has thickened to your desired consistency.

6. Decant the ketchup into a sterilized jar and store in the fridge for up to 3 weeks.

7. Add to *everything*!

Simple but Oh-So-Tasty Pasta Sauce

Yields: 4 cups

Ingredients:

4 pounds ripe tomatoes, chopped

1 cup basil leaves, chopped

3 tablespoons olive oil

8 garlic cloves, chopped

1 jalapeño pepper, finely chopped

1 teaspoon apple cider vinegar

1 tablespoon honey

Directions:

1. Heat the olive oil in a saucepan over a medium heat and then add the garlic and jalapeños. Sauté until just starting to brown, then add the tomatoes.
2. Bring the tomatoes to a boil, then reduce the heat and allow to simmer until the mixture has reduced by half. This takes about an hour, so be patient.
3. Now add the remaining ingredients to the pot and stir them in well.
4. Allow to simmer for a further 15 minutes, then decant into sterilized jars and refrigerate.
5. Alternatively, you can make a big batch and freeze the sauce for an easy go-to meal in a hurry.
6. Enjoy!

Mayonnaise

While store-bought mayonnaise might be convenient, it is packed full of unhealthy ingredients that are simply just not good for you. This homemade mayonnaise is quick and easy to make, is packed full of healthy goodness, and tastes fantastic to boot!

Yields: 4 servings

Ingredients:

1 cup olive oil
1 cup macadamia oil
5 egg yolks, at room
    temperature

1 tablespoon organic apple
    cider vinegar
1 tablespoon Dijon mustard
Salt and pepper to taste

Directions:

1. Add everything to the blender except for the oils and blend until well incorporated.
2. Now very slowly, a drop at a time, add the olive oil, while the blender runs continuously.
3. Keep adding the olive oil slowly until it starts to emulsify, then add the macadamia oil and keep blending until it is all incorporated.
4. Store in the fridge for 1 week.

Spicy Fruit Chutney

Yields: about 3 cups

Ingredients:

1 pound fresh apricots, pitted and chopped

2 cups dried apricots, sliced thinly

½ cup organic apple cider vinegar

½ cup rapadura

2 mangoes, pitted, peeled and chopped

4 garlic cloves, chopped

1 red chili pepper—finely diced

Zest of 1 lime, finely grated

1 tablespoon freshly grated ginger

1 teaspoon cinnamon

½ teaspoon cumin seeds

½ teaspoon mustard seeds

¼ teaspoon ground cloves

Directions:

1. Throw all the ingredients into a large pot and bring them to a boil over a medium heat.
2. Once boiling reduce the heat to low and simmer for an hour or until most of the liquid has evaporated. Stir the mixture frequently during the cooking time.
3. Once cooked, cover the pot and leave it overnight.
4. In the morning, reheat the pot, then ladle the chutney into a sterilized jar.

5. Leave the jar at room temperature for a week so the flavors meld and develop and then pop it into the fridge until needed.
6. Serve as a side to meat and cheese or as a part of a ploughman's lunch—enjoy!

Simple Herby Garlic Salad Dressing

Yields: about 2 cups

Ingredients:

1 ½ cups olive oil

½ cup organic apple cider
  vinegar

¼ cup fresh herbs of your
  choice

4 garlic cloves, minced

3 tablespoons Dijon mustard

Salt and black pepper to taste

Directions:

1. Throw it all in a jar.
2. Close the lid.
3. Shake to combine.
4. Pour over salad.

2 Shakes Vinaigrette

Yields: about 1 cup

Ingredients:

½ cup olive oil

¼ cup organic apple cider
    vinegar

2 garlic cloves, minced

2 tablespoons honey

2 tablespoons Dijon mustard

2 tablespoons lemon juice

Directions:

1. Place all the ingredients in a jar and shake to combine.
2. Store in the fridge for a week.
3. Shake well before serving.
4. Enjoy over your favorite salad greens.
5. Simple and tasty.

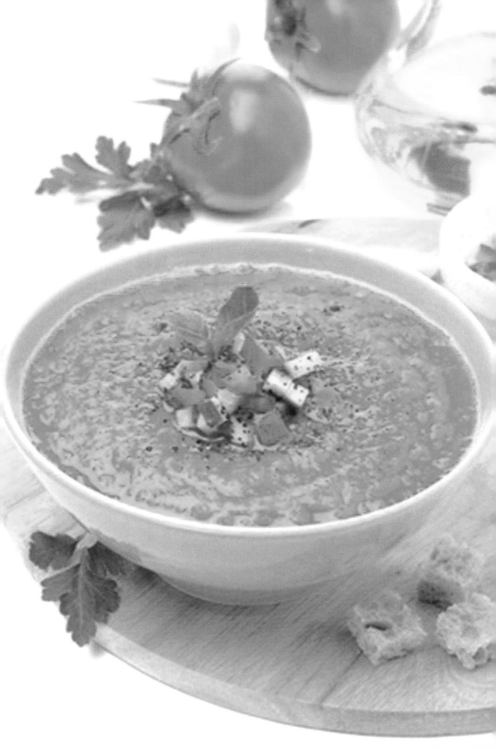

Soups

Quick Gazpacho

Using tomato juice instead of fresh tomatoes makes this a healthy, low-calorie treat that is easy to make.

Yields: 4 servings

Ingredients:

1 quart organic tomato juice

1 cucumber, seeded and chopped

1 green bell pepper, seeded and chopped

½ an onion, chopped

3 stalks celery, chopped

¼ cup organic apple cider vinegar

2 tablespoons tomato paste

1 tablespoon organic Worcestershire sauce

1 tablespoon chopped fresh parsley

1 teaspoon vegetable broth powder

½ teaspoon onion salt

¼ teaspoon freshly ground black pepper

¼ teaspoon garlic powder

Directions:

1. Process all the ingredients in several batches in a food processor or blender until smooth, using water to achieve your desired consistency.
2. Combine in a large bowl or pitcher, and refrigerate until chilled.
3. Serve and enjoy!

Bacon, Pumpkin, and Apple Soup

Yields: 4 servings

Ingredients:

15 ounces pumpkin puree

3 ½ cups organic or homemade vegetable stock

1 cup onions, chopped

½ cup apple juice, unsweetened

¼ cup coconut cream

1 apple, peeled, cored and diced small

6 slices bacon, chopped

4 garlic cloves, minced

2 tablespoons roasted pumpkin seeds

2 tablespoons organic apple cider vinegar

1 tablespoon butter

1 tablespoon maple syrup

1 teaspoon cinnamon

½ teaspoon nutmeg

½ teaspoon pumpkin pie spice

Directions:

1. Place the chopped bacon into a large soup pot and cook over a high heat until crispy. Remove with a slotted spoon to a paper towel lined plate and leave the bacon drippings in the pot.
2. Add the chopped onions to the bacon drippings and sauté over a medium heat for about 5 minutes or until they are soft, then add the garlic and cook for a further 2 minutes.

3. Pour in the stock, apple juice, pumpkin puree, pumpkin pie spice, cinnamon, and nutmeg and bring to a boil.
4. Once boiling, reduce the heat to low, add the chopped bacon back to the pot and allow to simmer for about 20 minutes.
5. When the soup is cooked, use an immersion blender to puree it until smooth and then stir in the coconut cream and apple cider vinegar.
6. Keep the soup over a low heat until it is warmed through and you are ready to serve it.
7. While the soup cooks, make the apples. Place the apples, butter, and maple syrup into a saucepan and cook over a medium heat until the apples are soft and brown, about 15 minutes.
8. To serve: ladle the soup into bowls and spoon a little of the apple on top, then garnish with roasted pumpkin seeds.
9. Grab a spoon and tuck in!

Onion Soup

Yields: 4 servings

Ingredients:

6 cups red onions, sliced

6 cups yellow onions, sliced

6 cups organic or homemade
beef broth

2 cups croutons (optional)

2 cups shredded cheese of your
choice (optional)

2 tablespoons olive oil

2 tablespoons organic butter

2 tablespoons organic apple
cider vinegar

1 tablespoon minced garlic

1 tablespoon chopped chives

Directions:

1. Heat up the olive oil and butter in a large pot, add the onions, cover and cook over a low heat for 1 hour, stirring every 10 minutes.

2. Remove the lid and cook for a further 30 minutes or until they are golden and caramelized, then add the garlic and sauté a further 5 minutes.

3. Add 2 cups of the beef broth and simmer, using a wooden spoon to scrape up all the browned bits off the bottom of the pan.

4. Now add the rest of the beef broth and simmer for an additional 15 minutes.

5. Use an immersion blender to puree the soup until it is smooth and creamy.

6. This step is optional: ladle the soup into 4 oven-safe bowls and place them onto a large baking tray. Top each bowl with some shredded cheese and croutons and pop the tray under the broiler until the cheese is melted and bubbly and the croutons are brown, about 2 minutes.

7. Remove from the oven and sprinkle over some chopped chives for garnish

Sweet Potato Soup

Yields: 4 servings

Ingredients:

4 cups organic or homemade
  vegetable broth
4 cups sweet potato, peeled and
  cubed
1 cup onion, chopped
1 cup carrots, peeled and
  chopped
½ cup low fat milk

1 tablespoon olive oil
1 tablespoon cumin
1 tablespoon organic apple
  cider vinegar
1 teaspoon curry powder
1 teaspoon fresh ginger, grated
1 teaspoon red pepper flakes

Directions:

1. Heat up the olive oil in a large pot, then sauté the onions until they begin to soften.
2. Add the carrots and sweet potato cubes and cook for a further 5 minutes, stirring gently and often so that the sweet potato does not stick.
3. Add the spices, apple cider vinegar, and vegetable broth and bring the pot to a boil.
4. Once boiling, reduce the heat and stir in the milk.
5. Cover and allow to simmer for 20 minutes.

6. Remove from the heat and use an immersion blender to puree until the soup is smooth and creamy.
7. Ladle into soup bowls and sprinkle with some red pepper flakes for garnish.
8. Enjoy!

Mushroom and Thyme Soup

Yields: 4 servings

Ingredients:

16 ounces of mushrooms, try to get a variety for a more complex flavor

1 onion, chopped

4 cups organic or homemade vegetable broth

¼ cup celery, chopped

4 garlic cloves, minced

1 tablespoon olive oil

1 tablespoon fresh thyme, chopped

1 tablespoon coconut aminos

1 tablespoon organic apple cider vinegar

1 tablespoon Worcestershire sauce

Salt and freshly ground black pepper to taste

Directions:

1. Heat up the olive oil in a large pot over a medium heat and then add the onions, mushrooms, and garlic. Sauté for 5 minutes or until the onions turn translucent.
2. Add the remaining ingredients except for the thyme, bring to a boil, then reduce the heat and simmer for about 30 minutes.
3. Use an immersion blender to puree the soup until it is smooth and creamy.
4. Ladle the soup into serving bowls and garnish with some chopped thyme.
5. Serve hot—delicious!

Pork and Cabbage Soup

Yields: 8 servings

Ingredients:

1 quart organic or homemade
    vegetable broth
1 pound cabbage, shredded
1 sweet potato, peeled and
    diced
1 parsnip, peeled and diced
8 ounces pork sausage, casings
    removed and crumbled
4 ounces smoked ham, diced
2 cups water

1 cup carrots, diced
1 onion, chopped
2 tablespoons organic apple
    cider vinegar
2 tablespoons celery, chopped
1 tablespoon paprika
1 teaspoon dried marjoram
4 garlic cloves, minced
2 bay leaves
Salt and black pepper to taste

Directions:

1. Brown the sausage meat in a large pot over a medium heat. Remove the sausage with a slotted spoon and set aside on a paper towel-lined plate to drain. Leave the sausage drippings in the pot.
2. Add the onion, celery, ham, garlic, carrots, salt, pepper, marjoram, and bay leaves to the pot and sauté until the onions are translucent.

3. Add the remaining ingredients and bring to a boil, then reduce the heat and allow to simmer for 30 minutes or until the potatoes and parsnips are tender.
4. Ladle into bowls and enjoy hot!

Spicy Carrot Soup

Yields: 4 servings

Ingredients:

1 pound carrots, chopped
½ pound sweet potato, chopped
4 cups organic or homemade
    vegetable broth
2 cups water
1 onion, quartered
4 garlic cloves, minced
2 tablespoons olive oil

2 tablespoons turmeric
2 tablespoons organic apple
    cider vinegar
1 tablespoon curry powder
1 tablespoon masala
1 teaspoon fresh ginger, grated
¼ teaspoon cayenne pepper

Directions:

1. Place 3 of the 4 onion quarters, carrots, and sweet potatoes onto a baking tray, drizzle with olive oil, season with salt and pepper, and bake in a 400°F oven for 30 minutes.
2. At the 20 minute mark, throw in the garlic cloves to roast as well.
3. Heat up some olive oil in a large pot over a medium heat.
4. Chop the remaining quarter of an onion and add it to the oil, along with all the spices and ginger and cook until the onion is soft.

5. Add the water, apple cider vinegar, and vegetable broth to the pot and bring to a boil, then turn down the heat and simmer gently.
6. Add the roasted veggies and garlic to the pot now, turn off the heat and allow it to cool down a bit.
7. Use an immersion blender to puree the soup until it is smooth and creamy.
8. Ladle into serving bowls and garnish with some cayenne pepper.
9. You can serve this soup with a dollop of low fat Greek yogurt too—delicious!

Slow Cooker Chicken Soup

Yields: 4–6 servings

Ingredients:

4 chicken breasts, bone in, skin on

4 chicken thighs, bone in, skin on

4 cups water

2 cups organic or homemade chicken broth

1 cup carrots, diced

1 onion, chopped

¼ cup celery, chopped

2 garlic cloves, minced

2 tablespoons fresh herbs, chopped

1 tablespoon organic apple cider vinegar

Salt and pepper to taste

Directions:

1. Layer all the vegetables into the slow cooker and then place the chicken, bone side down, on top.
2. Add the seasonings, garlic, and apple cider vinegar, then pour over the chicken broth.
3. Lastly add the water, cover, and cook on low for 6–8 hours.
4. Remove the chicken and allow it to cool down.
5. Debone the chicken and remove the skin, then shred the meat and add it back to the slow cooker.
6. Reheat and serve.
7. YUM!

Hearty Veggie Soup

Yields: 4–6 servings

Ingredients:

8 cups water, as needed

2 cups carrots, chopped

2 cups parsnips, chopped

2 cups sweet potato, peeled and cubed

1 cup beet, chopped

1 cup onion, chopped

½ cup organic apple cider vinegar

¼ cup celery, chopped

2 tablespoons olive oil

Fresh herbs of your choice

Salt and pepper to taste

Directions:

1. Heat up the olive oil in a large soup pot and sauté the onions until soft and translucent.
2. Add the rest of the vegetables and toss to coat with the onions and oil, then pour in enough water to cover the vegetables.
3. Bring the pot to a boil, then reduce the heat and allow it to simmer until the vegetables are tender.
4. Remove the pot from the heat, stir in the apple cider vinegar and some salt and pepper.
5. Serve hot!

Tomato Soup

Yields: 6 servings

Ingredients:

28 ounces diced tomatoes
28 ounces organic or
  homemade vegetable broth
15 ounces tomato sauce, preferably homemade
2 onions, chopped
4 garlic cloves, minced

1 tablespoon olive oil
1 tablespoon dried oregano
1 tablespoon organic apple
  cider vinegar
1 teaspoon rapadura
Salt and pepper to taste

Directions:

1. Heat up the olive oil in a large soup pot and sauté the onions until they are soft and translucent, then add the garlic and the tomatoes. Continue to cook until the tomatoes have broken down.
2. Now add the remaining ingredients and stir together well.
3. Bring to a boil, then reduce the heat and simmer for 20 minutes or until the soup has thickened slightly.
4. If you don't mind a chunky soup, serve as is, otherwise puree the soup first with an immersion blender.
5. Tasty!

Refreshing Apple Cider Soup

Yields: 4–6 servings

Ingredients:

4 cups unsweetened apple juice
4 cups organic or homemade
    chicken broth
2 apples, peeled, cored, and
    chopped

2 tablespoons apple cider
    vinegar
1 teaspoon ginger powder
Red pepper flakes to taste, for
    garnish

Directions:

1. Add everything to a large pot and bring it to a boil, then reduce the heat and allow the soup to simmer until the apples are soft.
2. Once the apples are soft, use an immersion blender to puree the apples into the liquid.
3. Ladle into soup bowls and garnish with a sprinkling of red pepper flakes.
4. Warm and cleansing—enjoy!

Tangy Parsnip Soup

Yields: 4 servings

Ingredients:

2 apples, peeled, cored and
diced

2 parsnips, peeled and sliced

1 sweet potato, peeled and
sliced

2 cups organic or homemade
vegetable stock

½ cup organic apple cider
vinegar

½ cup low fat milk (or
substitute coconut milk)

4 strips of bacon, cooked crispy
and crumbled

2 tablespoons low fat Greek
yogurt

Directions:

1. Place the apples, sweet potato, parsnips, apple cider
   vinegar, and stock into a large pot and bring to a
   gentle simmer.
2. Allow to cook until the apples, parsnips, and potato
   are tender.
3. Use an immersion blender to puree the soup until it
   is smooth and creamy and then stir in the milk and
   yogurt.
4. Place the pot over a low heat until it is warmed through
   and then ladle into bowls, topping with crumbled
   bacon for garnish.
5. Absolutely amazing!

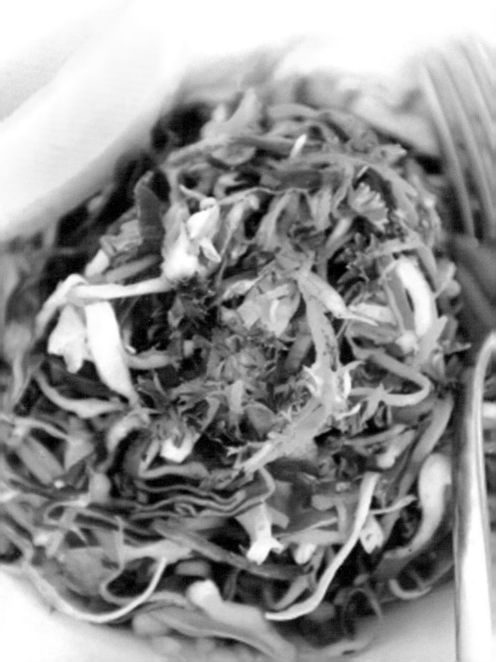

Salads

Sweet and Sour Slaw

Yields: 10 servings

Ingredients:

1 medium cabbage, shredded
(use a mix of red and white
cabbage)
1 large onion, finely diced
2 carrots, shredded
1 (4-ounce) jar diced pimentos
1 cup organic apple cider
vinegar

¼ cup golden raisins
½ cup olive oil
¼ cup raw organic honey
1 teaspoon turmeric
½ teaspoon salt

Directions:

1. Combine the cabbage, onion, carrots, and pimentos in a large bowl.
2. Mix the vinegar, olive oil, honey, turmeric, and salt in a jar, put on the lid, and shake well.
3. Pour the mixture over the vegetables, add the raisins, and toss lightly.
4. Serve immediately.

Kale and Avocado Salad

Kale is one of the highest scoring antioxidant foods on the ORAC scale.

Yields: 2 Servings

Ingredients:

1 bunch organic kale, stems
    removed
1 avocado, cut into bite-sized
    cubes
8 ounces organic cherry
    tomatoes, halved
¼ cup red onion, sliced

¼ cup sunflower seeds
1 tablespoon raw honey
1 tablespoon olive oil
¼ cup organic apple cider
    vinegar
Pinch of sea salt
Juice of ½ a lemon

Directions:

1. Tear the kale into bite-sized pieces and place them into a large salad bowl.
2. Prepare the vinaigrette by blending the honey, olive oil, vinegar, salt, and lemon juice in a blender until well combined.
3. Pour the vinaigrette over the kale and massage well until the kale has softened.
4. Top with the avocado cubes, red onion, cherry tomatoes, and sunflower seeds.
5. Serve immediately and enjoy!

Colorful Vegetable Slaw

Slaws that have other vegetable ingredients are both aesthetically appealing as well as high in nutritional value. Try this tasty slaw for something different!

Yields: 6–8 servings

Ingredients:

5 cups green cabbage, shredded

2 cups red cabbage, shredded

2 cups broccoli florets, finely chopped

½ cup cauliflower florets, finely chopped

8 green beans, sliced thin

1 red pepper, sliced thin

1 green pepper, sliced thin

1 onion, sliced thin

Dressing:

½ cup olive oil

¼ cup organic apple cider vinegar

2 teaspoons Dijon mustard

1 teaspoon raw organic honey

½ teaspoon sea salt

Directions:

1. Combine all the vegetables in a bowl.
2. Mix the dressing ingredients together well, pour over the vegetables, and toss.
3. Refrigerate for a few hours before serving.
4. Delicious!

Pear Salad

This unusual salad is the perfect opening act for a truly memorable meal.

Yields: 4 servings

Ingredients:

2 cups arugula

2 cups watercress

4 ripe pears

1 avocado

4 tablespoons sundried tomatoes, chopped

Dressing

½ cup olive oil

3 tablespoons organic apple cider vinegar

2 tablespoons raw organic honey

¼ teaspoon sea salt

1 tablespoon tomato paste

Directions:

1. Wash and remove the stems from the watercress and arugula and divide the greens up between 4 salad bowls.
2. Combine the dressing ingredients and set aside.
3. Peel the pears and avocado and slice them thinly. (Place the slices in some cold, salted water to prevent

discoloration if it will be a little while before you're ready to serve the salad.)

4. Rinse the pear and avocado slices well, and arrange them over the greens in the salad bowls.

5. Sprinkle 1 tablespoon of chopped sundried tomatoes over each bowl.

6. Add the dressing and serve immediately.

7. Scrumptious!

German Potato Salad

This traditional favorite comes from an old Mennonite recipe.

Yields: 8 servings

Ingredients:

4 pounds potatoes (about 8 cups sliced)

3 cups onion, chopped

¾ cup organic apple cider vinegar

¾ cup hot water

¼ cup organic bacon, cooked and diced

2 tablespoons raw organic honey or maple syrup

2 tablespoons chives, chopped

Sea salt and pepper to taste

Directions:

1. Boil the potatoes until tender.
2. Peel and slice them while warm.
3. Add the onions, honey, or maple syrup, bacon, salt, and pepper and toss gently.
4. Mix the apple cider vinegar mixed with the hot water, then pour the mixture over the potatoes, bacon, and onions.
5. Toss together lightly so as not to break up the potatoes too much.
6. Sprinkle with the chopped chives for garnish.
7. This salad can be served warm or cold—either way it is delicious!

Mixed Marinated Beans

This is a great dish for potluck dinners or to have on hand for suppers during the hot summer months. These beans are the perfect accompaniment to barbequed meat or a selection of cold meats.

Yields: 10 servings

Ingredients:

1 pound frozen green beans, cooked and drained

1 pound canned kidney beans, drained

1 pound canned wax beans, drained

1 onion, thinly sliced

1 green bell pepper, chopped

1 cup cherry tomatoes, sliced

¾ cup organic apple cider vinegar

¼ cup raw organic honey (optional)

½ cup olive oil

1 teaspoon garlic, minced

½ teaspoon salt

½ teaspoon freshly ground black pepper

Directions:

1. Combine the drained beans in a large bowl with the sliced onion, sliced cherry tomatoes, and bell peppers.
2. Mix the vinegar, honey, olive oil, garlic, salt, and black pepper in a jar, put the lid on and shake well.
3. Pour the mixture over the beans and toss well to combine.
4. Cover the bowl and marinate overnight in the refrigerator.
5. Serve when needed with your favorite meat dish.
6. YUM!

Rice Salad

Add some tofu or organic chicken to make a complete meal-in-a-bowl.

Yields: 4–6 servings

Ingredients:

1 cup brown rice, uncooked

2 cups water

1 cup green peas, cooked

1 cup asparagus tips, cooked

½ cup broccoli florets, cooked

½ cup green bell pepper, chopped

½ cup fresh parsley, chopped

¼ cup onion, finely chopped

¼ cup olive oil

3 tablespoons organic apple cider vinegar

2 tablespoons lemon juice

1 tablespoon fresh tarragon

Salt and pepper to taste

Cherry tomato halves, garnish

Green and/or black olives, garnish

Directions:

1. Simmer the brown rice in the water until just tender, about 30 minutes, then drain and place into a large salad bowl.
2. Immediately toss with the olive oil, apple cider vinegar, lemon juice, salt, pepper, tarragon, and onion, then set aside to cool.
3. Once cool, add the green pepper, parsley, peas, broccoli, and asparagus tips.

4. Toss gently to combine and chill in the fridge for a few hours.
5. Serve decorated with cherry tomato halves and sliced olives.
6. Very tasty.

Note: This is an incredibly versatile salad. This particular version is loaded with delicious crunchy greens, but you could just as easily substitute in your favorite selection of fresh veggies for a different taste every time. Have fun experimenting!

Variation: Add ½ pound cubed and cooked organic chicken or sautéed tofu.

Couscous Salad

Yields: 6 cups

Ingredients:

2 cups water

2 cups couscous

1 pound butternut squash, cut into strips

1 red pepper, seeds removed and cut into quarters

2 onions, peeled and quartered

¼ cup fresh parsley, chopped

3 tablespoons organic apple cider vinegar

6 tablespoons olive oil

3 tablespoons sesame seeds

1 tablespoon soy sauce

1 teaspoon garlic salt, or to taste

Salt and freshly ground black pepper to taste

Directions:

Toss the squash, red pepper, and onions with 3 tablespoons of olive oil and the garlic salt and roast in the oven at 350°F for 30 minutes or until they are tender and browning. Remove from the oven and set aside. When the veggies are cool enough to handle, you can chop the red pepper and onion up into bite sized pieces.

7. While the veggies roast, make the couscous. In a medium saucepan, bring the water to a boil, then stir

in the couscous. Cover, remove from the heat, and let stand for about 5 minutes or until all the water has been absorbed.

8. Combine the apple cider vinegar, salt, pepper, and soy sauce in a small bowl and set aside.

9. Sauté the sesame seeds in the remaining olive oil over a low heat for a minute or two until they just start to brown.

10. Remove from the heat. Add the vinegar and soy sauce mixture and stir together well.

11. Fluff the couscous lightly with a fork and break up any clumps.

12. Combine the couscous, roasted vegetables, and chopped parsley, then toss everything to mix.

13. Pour over the sesame seed, vinegar, and soy sauce mixture and toss again.

14. If you like, you can add a little more salt to taste and garnish with more chopped parsley.

15. Serve warm or chilled.

16. Out of this world!

Summer Salad with Poppy Seed Dressing

Yields: 2–4 servings

Ingredients:

8 ounces baby spinach leaves
2 avocados, diced
1 cup strawberries, sliced

¼ cup low fat feta cheese, crumbled
¼ cup slivered almonds

Dressing:

½ cup mayonnaise
¼ cup nonfat milk
2 tablespoons honey

2 tablespoons organic apple cider vinegar
2 teaspoons poppy seeds

Directions:

1. Combine all the salad ingredients in a large bowl and toss lightly to mix them up.
2. Whisk up the dressing ingredients in a jug until they are well combined.
3. Pour the dressing over the salad and serve immediately.
4. It doesn't get easier than this!

Quick Quinoa Salad

Yields: 2 servings

Ingredients:

2 cups quinoa, cooked and
cooled
½ cup golden raisins
½ cup dried cranberries
½ cup freshly chopped mint
1 red pepper, seeded and
chopped
1 yellow pepper, seeded and
chopped

1 red onion, chopped finely
¼ cup olive oil
¼ cup organic apple cider
vinegar
¼ cup freshly squeezed lemon
juice

Directions:

1. Toss everything together in a large bowl and make
sure it is all thoroughly combined.
2. Serve immediately.
3. Quick, easy, and very yummy!

Sweet Potato Salad

Yields: 4 servings

Ingredients:

4 sweet potatoes, peeled and diced

1 red onion, finely diced

¼ cup celery, finely diced

½–1 cup light mayonnaise

2 tablespoons fresh cilantro, chopped

1 tablespoon organic apple cider vinegar

1 tablespoon cumin

1 teaspoon curry powder

Juice of ½ a lemon

Zest of ½ a lemon

Salt and black pepper to taste

Directions:

1. Boil the sweet potatoes in some lightly salted water until they are fork tender, then drain and set aside to cool.
2. Mix the rest of the ingredients together in a bowl and pour over the potatoes.
3. Toss to coat well.
4. Serve with your favorite grilled meat. Amazing!

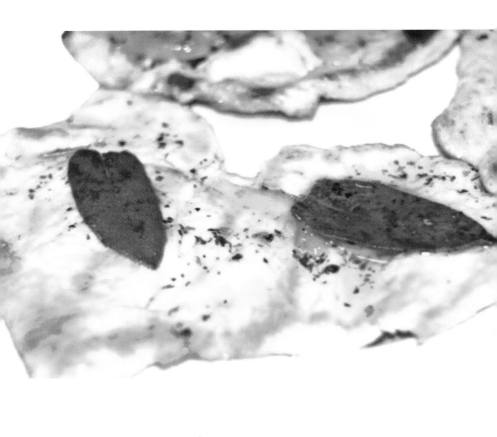

Main Meals and Side Dishes

Apple Cider Vinegar and Sage Chicken

Yields: 4 servings

Ingredients:

4 chicken breasts, bone in and skin on

2 cups organic chicken stock

1 ¼ cups organic apple cider vinegar

3 onions, thinly sliced

4 tablespoons extra virgin olive oil

3 tablespoons sage, chopped

3 tablespoons honey

4 garlic cloves, chopped

Juice of ½ a lemon

Salt and pepper to taste

Directions:

1. Preheat a Dutch oven over a medium-high heat.
2. Add two tablespoons of olive oil to the pan.
3. Season chicken with salt and pepper, then add them to the hot oil, skin side down.
4. Brown the chicken for about 5 minutes per side, then remove them from the pan and set them aside for later.
5. Add another 2 tablespoons of olive oil to the pan, then add the onion slices, sage, honey, and the garlic.

6. Season the onions with salt and pepper and cook over a medium-low heat, stirring frequently for about 20 minutes or until the onions are really brown and starting to caramelize.
7. Add the apple cider vinegar to deglaze the pan, taking care to scrape up all the brown bits on the bottom of the pan with a wooden spoon.
8. Now add the chicken stock and heat the mixture until it starts to bubble.
9. Once at a rolling simmer, return the chicken to the pot with the liquid and onions.
10. Place a lid on the pot, turn the heat to medium and simmer for about 20 minutes, turning the chicken over in the sauce about halfway through the cooking time.
11. When the 20 minutes is up, remove the lid and check to make sure the chicken is cooked through by cutting a small slit in the thickest part of the breast with a paring knife to have a look inside. If it is cooked through the juices will run clear and the meat will be white not pink.
12. Remove the chicken to a plate, squeeze over the lemon juice, and cover with foil to keep warm.
13. Turn the heat of the sauce up to high and simmer until the sauce thickens up slightly, about 4–5 minutes.
14. Serve the chicken drizzled with the sauce and your favorite side dish of vegetables or a healthy salad.
15. Dig in!

Roast Beef with Apple Cider Vinegar

Yields: 4–6 servings

Ingredients:

2 onions, sliced

3 tablespoons of olive oil

3 pound beef roast

1 cup organic apple cider vinegar

2 cups organic beef stock

6 garlic cloves, halved

6 garlic cloves, minced

Steak seasoning to taste

Directions:

1. Using a sharp paring knife, cut 12 deep slits in the beef roast, taking care to space them out more or less evenly.

2. Insert ½ a garlic clove into each one and push them in deep.

3. Massage the meat with the olive oil to tenderize and then rub in as much steak seasoning as you like.

4. Finally rub the minced garlic over the outside of the meat, cover and refrigerate for at least 2 hours prior to cooking to marinade and allow all the flavors to soak in.

5. When you are ready to cook the meat, layer some onion rings on the bottom of a lightly greased oven proof dish, place the beef on top of the onions and arrange the remaining onion slices over the meat.

6. In the meantime, combine the apple cider vinegar and beef stock and whisk them together well.

7. Pour the mixture over the beef, cover with foil or a lid, and put into a 325°F oven.

8. Cook the beef for about 3 hours or until tender.

9. Every hour or so, turn the beef in the cooking liquid.

10. When the beef is cooked to your taste, remove it carefully from the oven and set aside to rest for 10 minutes before carving.

11. While the meat rests, pour the cooking liquid and onions into a saucepan and using an immersion blender, purée until the onions have been incorporated into the cooking liquid. If the gravy is not thick enough, use your choice of thickener to achieve the desired consistency.

12. Slice the beef, pour over the gravy, and serve with your choice of side vegetables or salad.

13. Unbelievable!

Green Tomato Mincemeat

This is a great vegetarian substitute for traditional mincemeat and makes good use of any green tomatoes you may have left over at the end of gardening season. It's perfect for pies and in a decorated canning jar becomes a festive homemade gift.

Yields: 10 pints

Ingredients:

4 pounds apples (about 8 cups)

3 pounds green tomatoes (about 6 cups)

2 pounds raisins

2 pounds rapadura

1 ¼ cups organic apple cider vinegar

3 tablespoons cinnamon

3 tablespoons lemon juice

3 tablespoons orange juice

1 tablespoon finely grated orange zest

1 tablespoon finely grated lemon zest

2 teaspoons nutmeg

2 teaspoons sea salt

1 teaspoon ground cloves

Directions:

1. Mince the tomatoes up by grinding them in a food processor.
2. Add the salt and let this mixture stand for 1 hour.
3. Drain the tomatoes, place them in a pot, and add just enough water to cover them.

4. Bring the pot to a boil and cook for 5 minutes, then drain them again and set them aside for later.
5. Peel, core, and chop the apples up into small pieces.
6. Place them in a large, heavy-bottomed saucepan, then add the tomatoes and the remaining ingredients and mix it all together thoroughly.
7. Bring to a boil, then reduce the heat and simmer gently for 1 hour, stirring frequently.
8. When the hour is up, remove the pot from the heat and ladle the mixture into 10 hot, sterilized, pint canning jars and seal with sterilized canning lids.
9. Use when required.

Note: To make a pie with this, preheat the oven to 425°F. Fill an 8-inch pie crust with some of the cooled mixture and cover with a top crust. Prick the top or cut slits to allow steam to escape. Bake for 15 minutes, then reduce the heat to 375°F and continue baking for 35 minutes. Allow to cool slightly, slice, and serve.

Marinated Mushrooms

The combination of mushrooms with apple cider vinegar makes this appetizer especially high in potassium.

Yields: 10 servings

Ingredients:

½ cup organic apple cider
    vinegar
½ cup olive oil
4 tablespoons chopped fresh
    parsley
1 tablespoon fresh thyme,
    chopped

1 tablespoon salt
1 tablespoon raw honey
1 teaspoon prepared mustard
1 teaspoon garlic, minced
1 small onion, sliced
1 pound fresh button
    mushrooms

Directions:

1. Combine everything except the onions and mushrooms in a saucepan and bring it to a boil, then remove from the heat.
2. Add the onion slices and whole mushrooms, allow to come to room temperature and then refrigerate overnight.
3. Serve when desired.
4. Delicious!

Marinated Vegetables

This makes a wonderful party appetizer.

Yields: 10 servings

Have ready:

6–8 cups of a mixture of your favorite vegetables, cut into bite-size pieces. You can use cauliflower, artichoke hearts, olives, bell peppers, mushrooms, carrots, zucchini, or cucumber. Cherry tomatoes and red bell peppers are also nice additions for their color.

Marinade:

1 ½ cups olive oil
¾ cup organic apple cider vinegar
2 teaspoons salt

1 teaspoon freshly ground black pepper
2 cloves garlic, crushed
¼ cup rapadura

Directions:

1. Place all the veggies, except the cherry tomatoes, in a large bowl.
2. Mix the marinade ingredients, pour over the prepared vegetables, and refrigerate. There won't be enough marinade to cover the vegetables, but that's alright. Stir the mixture several times a day for 3 days so that

all the vegetables will be sitting in the marinade for some of the time.

3. Add the cherry tomatoes on the last day.
4. Before serving, remove the garlic cloves and drain the vegetables.
5. Serve with toothpicks.
6. Tasty!

Spinach with Quinoa and Chickpeas

Spinach is rich in chlorophyll, which helps to cleanse the blood and colon.

Yields: 2–4 servings

Ingredients:

1 cup organic baby spinach leaves

½ cup chickpeas, cooked

½ cup red quinoa, cooked

½ cup artichoke hearts, cooked

½ an avocado, cut into cubes

8 organic cherry tomatoes

1 tablespoon organic apple cider vinegar

3 tablespoons olive oil

1 tablespoon raw honey

1 teaspoon mustard powder

Directions:

1. To prepare the vinaigrette, blend the apple cider vinegar, olive oil, mustard powder, and honey with a whisk, then set aside.
2. Place the baby spinach in a large serving bowl and toss with the prepared vinaigrette.
3. Add the quinoa and toss until well incorporated.
4. Top with chickpeas, artichoke hearts, cherry tomatoes, and avocado.
5. Devour!

Sweet Potato Chili

Yields: 4 servings

Ingredients:

4 cups organic or homemade
  vegetable stock
2 cups pinto beans
2 cups sweet potatoes, cubed
1 cup baby spinach leaves,
  chopped
½ cup frozen corn
28 ounces diced tomatoes
1 onion, chopped
4 garlic cloves, minced
2 chilies, seeds removed and
  finely diced

2 tablespoons olive oil
1 tablespoon organic apple
  cider vinegar
1 tablespoon chili powder
1 tablespoon cumin
1 tablespoon fresh cilantro,
  chopped (garnish)
Juice of 1 lime
Salt and pepper to taste

Directions:

1. Heat the olive oil in a pot over a medium heat, then add the onions and garlic and cook until the onions are translucent.

2. Add the spices and cook for a few minutes until they are fragrant, then add the tomatoes and apple cider vinegar. Stir and cook until the tomatoes begin to break down.

3. Now add the beans, vegetable stock, and sweet potato. Allow to simmer gently until the sweet potato is soft but not falling apart, about 30 minutes.
4. Add the chopped spinach and corn and allow to cook for a further 10 minutes, then squeeze in the lime juice just before serving.
5. Season with salt and pepper and sprinkle over some chopped cilantro.
6. Delicious served with diced avocado and tortillas.
7. Dig in!

Battered Cauliflower with Tangy Tomato Dipping Sauce

Yields: 2 servings

Ingredients:

For the Batter:

¾ cup rice flour

¾ cup sparkling water

½ cup corn starch (or substitute tapioca)

¼ teaspoon baking soda

Pinch of salt

For the Sauce:

2 cups mixed peppers, chopped (red, green, yellow, and orange)

1 red onion, chopped

¼ cup cashews, roughly chopped

¼ cup tomato paste, no added sugar

4 tablespoons coconut aminos

4 tablespoons organic or homemade vegetable stock

2 tablespoons organic apple cider vinegar

1 tablespoon fresh ginger, grated

1 tablespoon garlic, minced

2 teaspoons Stevia

1 teaspoon sesame oil

1 teaspoon red pepper flakes

Other ingredients:

2 pounds cauliflower, cut into small florets

¾ cup rice flour

Directions:

1. Preheat the oven to 400°F.

2. First prepare your batter: mix all the batter ingredients together until they are smooth. Place in the fridge to chill.

3. Boil your cauliflower florets in some lightly salted water for about 5 minutes or until they are just beginning to soften. Drain and then pour cold water over them to stop the cooking process. Set them aside to cool.

4. Place the rice flour into a resealable bag and add the cooled cauliflower pieces. Gently shake the bag to coat the cauliflower in the rice flour.

5. Dip each floret into the chilled batter, then place the cauliflower onto a parchment lined baking tray and bake for 10 minutes, then turn them over and bake for another 10 minutes. The cauliflower is cooked when it has a crunchy golden crust.

6. Remove the cauliflower to a plate to cool down and make the sauce.

7. Heat up the sesame oil in a large non-stick pan and add the peppers, onion, ginger, and garlic. Cook until the onions and peppers are soft, then add the rest of the ingredients and stir together well.

8. Bring the sauce to a boil, stirring constantly, then remove from the heat and add the cauliflower.

9. Totally YUM!

Vegetarian Pad Thai

Yields: 2 servings

Ingredients:

For the "Pasta":
2 sweet potatoes, spiraled
2 carrots, julienned
1 red onion, thinly sliced
1 red pepper, thinly sliced
¼ cup raw cashews, roughly
  chopped
¼ cup organic or homemade
  vegetable stock
3 tablespoons cilantro, finely
  chopped
Salt and pepper to taste

For the Sauce:
2 tablespoons sriracha sauce
2 tablespoons almond milk
2 tablespoons peanut butter
1 tablespoon maple syrup
1 teaspoon sesame oil
1 teaspoon turmeric
1 teaspoon organic apple cider
  vinegar

Directions:

1. Place the carrots and sweet potatoes into a pot and add the vegetable stock. Cover and cook for 5 minutes, then add the onions and red pepper.
2. Cook until the veggies are tender crisp, then add the cashews and cook for 1 more minute.
3. Remove the pot from the heat and set aside.

4. Whisk all the sauce ingredients together and pour over your "pasta."
5. Toss to coat and sprinkle with the chopped cilantro.
6. Season with salt and pepper and serve.
7. Enjoy!

Broccoli Stir Fry

Yields: 4 servings

Ingredients:

4 cups broccoli florets
1 red onion, sliced
1 tablespoon sesame oil
1 teaspoon minced garlic

1 teaspoon organic apple cider
   vinegar
1 teaspoon honey
1 red chili, seeds removed and
   chopped

Directions:

1. Boil the broccoli until it is tender-crisp, then run it under cold water to stop the cooking process.
2. Heat up the sesame oil in a non-stick pan and sauté the onions until they are soft, then add the broccoli and toss in the oil to coat.
3. Whisk the rest of the ingredients together and pour into the pan.
4. Cook for about 5 minutes, until the sauce is reduced by half and the broccoli is cooked to your liking. Take care not to stir the pan too much as the broccoli will break up.
5. Serve with a bowl of wild rice for a complete vegetarian meal, or serve this as an accompaniment to your favorite meat dish.
6. Either way—enjoy it!

Loaded Spuds

Yields: 4 servings

Ingredients:

4 sweet potatoes

2 tangerines, peeled and
separated into segments

2 avocados, peeled, pitted and
diced

1 red onion, finely diced

½ cup feta cheese, crumbled

¼ cup cilantro leaves

3 tablespoons olive oil

3 tablespoons red onion, finely
diced

2 tablespoons organic apple
cider vinegar

1 tablespoon cilantro, finely
chopped

1 teaspoon finely grated ginger

¼ teaspoon cayenne pepper

Juice of 1 lime

Zest of 1 lime

Salt to taste

Directions:

1. Wash and dry the sweet potatoes. Poke holes into them
   with a fork. Cover the sweet potatoes in foil and bake
   for 1 hour in a 400° F oven.
2. While they cook, make the dressing. Whisk together
   the olive oil, 3 tablespoons of red onion, apple cider
   vinegar, finely chopped cilantro, ginger, cayenne
   pepper, lime juice, and lime zest.

3. When the sweet potatoes are cooked, remove them from the oven and unwrap them.
4. Cut each one three-quarters of the way through with a very sharp knife and pour in a drizzle of the dressing.
5. Now top each sweet potato with some red onion, avocado, feta cheese, and tangerine wedges, then top with some more dressing.
6. Finally finish off with a sprinkling of cilantro leaves.
7. Serve immediately.
8. Simply superb!

Filipino Chicken

Yields: 4 servings

Ingredients:

4 chicken thighs, skin on, bone in

4 chicken drumsticks, skin on, bone in

½ cup organic apple cider vinegar

½ cup water

½ cup soy sauce (or substitute coconut aminos)

¼ cup sweet chili sauce

1 tablespoon raw honey

8 garlic cloves, crushed

2 bay leaves

1 teaspoon black peppercorns, crushed

Salt to taste

Directions:

1. Mix all the ingredients together in a large pot and leave it overnight to marinade and absorb all the flavors.
2. When you are ready to cook the dish, simply put the pot on the stove and bring it to a boil over a medium low heat.
3. Once boiling, reduce the heat slightly and allow to cook for about 20 minutes with the lid on.
4. After 20 minutes, remove the lid and turn the chicken pieces over and simmer until the sauce reduces and

thickens, turning the chicken in the sauce to ensure even cooking.

5. Serve over a bed of wild rice or basmati rice.

6. Divine!

Tastes of Fall Chicken

Yields: 4 servings

Ingredients:

2 pounds chicken breasts, skinless, boneless

2 onions, peeled and quartered

2 apples, cored and quartered, peel on

4 slices bacon, chopped

2 cups organic or homemade chicken stock

1 cup apple cider

¼ cup organic apple cider vinegar

3 tablespoons plain flour

1 tablespoon fresh thyme, chopped

1 tablespoon olive oil

Salt to taste

Directions:

1. Place the chicken into a large bowl, season with salt and thyme, and pour the apple cider over it and set aside to marinade.

2. Heat up the olive oil in a non-stick pan and sauté the onion wedges and chopped bacon until they start to turn brown, then add the apple wedges and cook until they begin to soften around the edges. Remove from the pan and set aside

3. Remove the chicken pieces from the apple cider, but reserve the liquid. Sprinkle the chicken with the flour

and add it to the pan you cooked the apples, bacon, and onions in.

4. Brown the chicken on both sides, then add the apple cider vinegar, chicken stock, and reserved apple cider and bring to a boil.

5. Once boiling, reduce the heat and add the onions, apples, and bacon back to the pan.

6. Place the whole pan into a preheated oven at 350°F for about 15 minutes or until the chicken is cooked through.

7. Serve with your choice of sides or on a bed of rice or noodles.

8. Scrumptious!

Braised Chicken Thighs

Yields: 2 servings

Ingredients:

6 chicken thighs, bone in,
    skin on
2 cups organic or homemade
    chicken stock
½ cup organic apple cider
    vinegar
¼ cup celery, chopped
2 carrots, peeled and sliced

1 leek, sliced
1 onion, chopped
4 garlic cloves, minced
1 tablespoon butter
1 tablespoon olive oil
1 tablespoon plain flour
Salt and pepper to taste

Directions:

1. Heat the olive oil up in a Dutch oven, then place the chicken pieces in skin side down and cook until the skin is golden-brown and crispy.
2. Remove the chicken from the pot and drain off most of the oil, leaving about 1 tablespoon, then add the onions, carrots, celery, garlic, and leek and cook until they begin to soften, stirring often.
3. Stir in the flour and cook for a further 2 minutes, then deglaze the pan with the apple cider vinegar. Take care to scrape up all the bits of browned chicken

off the bottom of the pan, then pour in the stock and bring it all to a boil.

4. Once boiling, add the chicken back to the pot, skin side up.

5. Cover the Dutch oven and place it into a 350°F oven for 1 hour.

6. When the cooking time is up, place the chicken pieces onto a baking tray and pop them under the broiler so that the skin can crisp up again.

7. While the chicken cooks, place the pot onto the stove and allow the sauce to reduce and thicken over a medium heat, then stir in the butter.

8. Serve the chicken slathered in delicious sauce with your choice of sides.

9. Enjoy!

Corned Beef and Cabbage

Yields: 8 servings

Ingredients:

3 pounds corned beef brisket, cut in half

2 cabbages, cut into wedges

1 pound baby carrots

4 sweet potatoes, cut into wedges

2 onions, cut into wedges

3 cups water

¼ cup mustard

8 garlic cloves, chopped

1 bay leaf

2 tablespoons apple cider vinegar

1 tablespoon grated ginger

Salt and pepper to taste

Directions:

1. Place all the vegetables (except the cabbage) into the bowl of a slow cooker.
2. Rub the mustard over the beef and place it on top of the vegetables.
3. Lastly add the cabbage on top of the beef.
4. Mix the remaining ingredients together in a bowl, and pour into the slow cooker.
5. Cover and cook on low for 8 hours.
6. Serve.
7. A complete meal in a pot—what more could you ask for?

Steak on the Barbie

Yields: 2 servings

Ingredients:

1 pound rib eye steak
¾ cup organic apple cider
 vinegar
¼ cup low sodium soy sauce
1 teaspoon raw honey

1 teaspoon grated ginger
3 garlic cloves, crushed
Salt and pepper to taste
Olive oil to drizzle

Directions:

1. Place the steak in a resealable plastic bag with the apple cider vinegar, soy sauce, honey, ginger, and crushed garlic. Give the bag a gentle shake to mix everything together and place it into the fridge to marinade for 2 hours.
2. When you are ready to cook the steak, remove it from the bag, sprinkle it with salt and pepper to taste and a little drizzle of olive oil.
3. Fire up the BBQ and place your steak onto the grill when it is hot—the steak should sizzle when it touches the grill.
4. Cook for about 4 minutes per side for medium rare. Adjust the times for your desired level of doneness.

5. Remove from the grill and cover with a tent of foil to rest for 10 minutes.
6. In the meantime, heat up the marinade in a saucepan over a medium high heat and allow to boil for about 5 minutes.
7. Slice the steak and dip it in the sauce.
8. Serve with your choice of side salad.
9. Enjoy!

Pork Tenderloin

Yields: 4–6 servings

Ingredients:

4 pounds pork tenderloin

2 cups unsweetened apple juice

½ cup Dijon mustard

4 garlic cloves, minced

4 tablespoons olive oil

2 tablespoons organic apple cider vinegar

2 tablespoons fresh sage

2 tablespoons butter

Salt and pepper to taste

Directions:

1. Preheat your oven to 375°F.
2. Season your tenderloin to taste with pepper and salt.
3. Heat up the olive oil in a large skillet set over a medium high heat until it starts to smoke.
4. Sear the tenderloin on all sides for about two minutes each.
5. Turn the heat off and move the tenderloin to a shallow baking pan.
6. Place the pork in the oven to roast until the internal temperature has reached 145 °F this should take approximately thirty minutes.
7. While the tenderloin is roasting use the same skillet as before, set to a high heat, to cook the garlic. Cook

for thirty seconds then add the apple cider vinegar, the apple juice, the Dijon mustard, and the sage.

8. Cook until the sauce starts to thicken and has reduced by at least two-thirds. Now turn the heat off and whisk the cold butter in until completely melted. Season to taste.

9. When the tenderloin is done remove it from the oven and set it on the cutting board, allow it to rest for at least ten minutes before slicing.

10. Serve with the warm sauce.

Slow Cooked Pot Roast

Yields: 8 servings

Ingredients:

3 pounds beef roast
¼ cup organic apple cider
   vinegar
¼ cup Worcestershire sauce

1 tablespoon minced garlic
1 tablespoon dried oregano
Salt and pepper to taste
Water as needed

Directions:

1. Rub the roast all over with the garlic and add it to the slow cooker.
2. Mix the rest of the ingredients together and pour into the slow cooker.
3. Add enough water so that it comes about half way up the meat.
4. Cover and cook on low for 8 hours.
5. Remove the roast and allow it to rest for 10 minutes before carving.
6. Pour some of the broth from the slow cooker over the meat once it is sliced.
7. Serve with your choice of sides.
8. Absolutely amazing!

Braised Pork Casserole

Yields: 4 servings

Ingredients:

2 ½ pounds pork shoulder, trimmed of excess fat and cut into cubes

2 onions, chopped

2 cups unsweetened apple juice

¾ cup organic apple cider vinegar

2 tablespoons olive oil

2 tablespoons fresh sage, chopped

1 tablespoon butter

2 bay leaves

2 garlic cloves, minced

Salt and pepper to taste

Directions:

1. Place an oven-proof casserole dish over a high heat on the stove. Add half the butter and half the oil and brown the pork in batches, placing them onto a plate when they are done.
2. Add the rest of the butter and the oil and brown the onions and garlic.
3. Pour the apple juice and apple cider vinegar into the pan to deglaze, carefully scraping all the browned bits off the bottom of the pan with a wooden spoon.
4. Place the pork back into the pan along with the rest of the ingredients and bring it to a simmer.

5. Once simmering, place the whole dish into an oven preheated to 325°F and cook uncovered for 1 hour or until the meat is tender and the cooking liquid has reduced.
6. Serve hot with some rice.
7. Delicious!

Roast Pork and Apples

Yields: 6 servings

Ingredients:

For the Pork:

4 pound pork loin roast, bone in

2 onions, sliced thick

2 cups organic or homemade vegetable stock

4 garlic cloves, crushed

2 tablespoons rosemary, chopped

2 tablespoons honey

2 tablespoons organic apple cider vinegar

Salt to taste

For the Apples:

6 apples, cored

¼ cup butter

¼ cup gluten free bread crumbs

1 onion, finely chopped

Zest of 1 lemon

Juice of 1 lemon

1 tablespoon freshly chopped rosemary

Directions:

1. Mix the salt, rosemary, and garlic together in a bowl. Make some deep cuts in the pork and rub the mixture all over the meat, taking care to push some into the slits.

2. Preheat the oven to 400° F. place the onions into a roasting pan and place the pork roast on top. Cover with foil and roast for 30 minutes.

3. Reduce the oven temperature to 350°F and bake for a further hour, then remove the foil and cook uncovered for 30 minutes.

4. Now prepare the apples—melt the butter in a saucepan and sauté the onions until they are soft.

5. Remove the pan from the heat and stir in the breadcrumbs, rosemary, lemon zest, and juice.

6. Fill the cored apples with the onion stuffing.

7. Now whisk the honey and apple cider vinegar together for the glaze.

8. Remove the pork from the oven and place the apples around the meat. Brush the meat with some of the glaze and pour the rest over the apples.

9. Place the whole roasting pan back into the oven and cook for a further 30 minutes or until the pork juices run clear when pierced with a fork.

10. Once cooked, place the apples and pork onto a plate, cover with foil and allow to rest for 10 minutes.

11. Meanwhile, place the roasting pan over a high heat on the stove and pour in the stock.

12. Bring to a boil, adding a little more honey and apple cider vinegar to taste if desired.

13. Slice the pork and serve with the stuffed apples and honey cider sauce drizzled over.

14. Out of this world!

Apple Cider Vinegar Pork Chops

Yields: 6 servings

Ingredients:

6 pork chops

2 cups unsweetened apple juice

¼ cup organic apple cider vinegar

¼ cup finely chopped onion

1 tablespoon olive oil

1 tablespoon butter

1 tablespoon Dijon mustard

1 tablespoon minced sage

¼ teaspoon red pepper flakes

4 garlic cloves, minced

Salt and pepper to taste

Directions:

1. Heat the oil and butter in a large non-stick pan over a medium heat and brown the pork chops on both sides. Transfer the pork chops to a plate.
2. Now add the onion and garlic to the pan and cook until they start to brown.
3. Now pour in the apple juice and apple cider vinegar and scrape up all the browned bits with a wooden spoon.
4. Add the mustard, stir, and bring to a boil.
5. Once boiling, reduce the heat and cook until the sauce thickens, about 5 minutes.

6. Stir in the rosemary and red pepper flakes, then return the chops to the pan and heat them through.
7. Season with salt and pepper and then serve with your favorite side dish.
8. Enjoy!

Easy Beef Stew

Yields: 6 servings

Ingredients:

3 pounds beef stew meat, cubed

1 pound baby potatoes, halved

6 carrots, sliced

3 celery stalks, sliced

2 onions, diced

1 apple, sliced

3 cups organic or homemade beef stock

1 cup water

¼ cup organic apple cider vinegar

3 tablespoons olive oil

3 tablespoons flour

1 tablespoon dried oregano

1 bay leaf

6 garlic cloves, crushed

Salt and black pepper to taste

Directions:

1. Mix the flour, oregano, salt, and pepper in a bowl and toss the beef cubes with the mixture.
2. Heat the oil in a large pot and brown the beef cubes in batches over a medium heat.
3. Add the beef stock, water, and apple cider vinegar to the beef cubes and bring the pot to a boil.
4. Add the bay leaf and garlic and reduce the heat to low.

5. Cook for 1 hour, then add the rest of the ingredients and simmer for a further hour or until all the vegetables are tender.
6. Serve with rice.
7. Delicious!

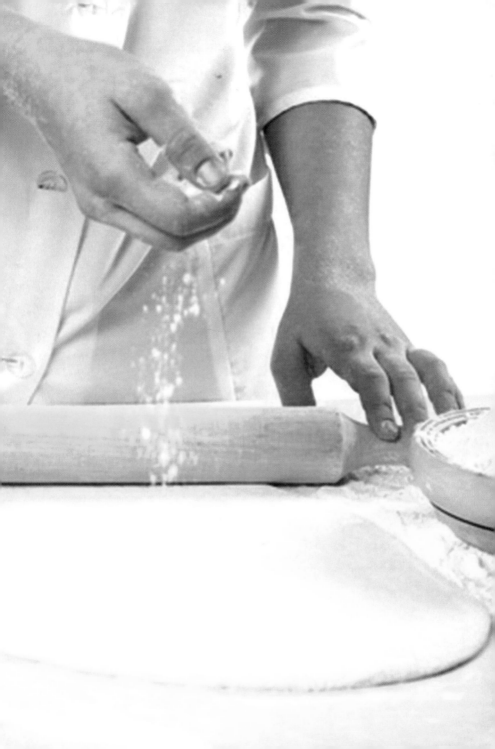

Desserts

Easy Apple Cider Vinegar Pastry Dough

Yields: dough for 2 crusts

Ingredients:

2 cups sifted organic spelt flour
¾ cup organic butter
2 tablespoons organic apple
    cider vinegar

2 tablespoons organic milk
1 teaspoon salt

Directions:

1. Combine the flour and salt in a mixing bowl, then cut in the butter with a pastry blender or two knives until the mixture looks crumbly and is about the size of small peas.
2. Sprinkle over the vinegar, then the milk, and gather up the flour mixture gently until it just holds together. Do not handle the dough any more than is necessary.
3. Roll it out and use it as a pie crust.
4. Add your favorite pie filling.
5. Bake, slice, EAT!

Chocolate Cake

Yields: 1 (9-inch) cake

Ingredients:

1 ½ cups organic white spelt
  flour

1 cup rapadura

1 cup cold water

⅓ cup olive oil

¼ cup cocoa powder

2 eggs

1 tablespoon organic apple
  cider vinegar

1 teaspoon baking soda

1 teaspoon vanilla

½ teaspoon salt

Directions:

1. Preheat the oven to 350°F.
2. Combine the flour, rapadura, cocoa, baking soda, and salt in a medium mixing bowl.
3. Add the apple cider vinegar, vanilla, oil, and cold water and beat until smooth.
4. Pour into a 9-inch square baking pan and bake for 30 to 35 minutes or until a toothpick inserted in the middle comes out clean.
5. Cool completely on a wire rack before frosting.
6. Frost, slice, and serve!
7. Store any leftovers in an airtight container.

Apple Cider Vinegar Pie

This is a basic recipe for "transparent" pie that's a Southern regional favorite.

Yields: 1 (8-inch) pie

Ingredients:

1 ½ cups organic sugar

½ cup organic apple cider vinegar

¼ cup organic flour

2 egg yolks

2 cups water

1 tablespoon melted butter

½ teaspoon lemon extract

1 (8-inch) unbaked pie crust

Directions:

1. Preheat the oven to 450°F.
2. Beat the egg yolks, water, apple cider vinegar, and melted butter together.
3. Mix the flour and sugar together, then stir it into the vinegar mixture.
4. Add the lemon extract and pour the mixture carefully into the unbaked pie shell.
5. Bake for 10 minutes, then reduce the heat to 350°F and continue to bake for a further 20 to 30 minutes or until a toothpick inserted into the edge of the pie comes out clean.
6. Cool completely before slicing and serving.
7. Delicious!

Holiday Pie

This variation of traditional vinegar pie is festive enough for the holidays.

Yields: 1 (8-inch) pie

Ingredients:

2 eggs

1 cup rapadura

½ cup chopped nuts of your choice (pistachios are a festive choice)

½ cup cranberries

½ cup shredded coconut

½ cup butter or nondairy spread suitable for baking

1 teaspoon vanilla

1 teaspoon organic apple cider vinegar

1 (8-inch) unbaked pie crust

Directions:

1. Preheat the oven to 325°F.
2. Mix the eggs, butter, and rapadura together.
3. Add the vanilla and apple cider vinegar, then fold in the nuts, cranberries, and coconut.
4. Pour into the unbaked pie crust and bake for 45 minutes.
5. Allow to cool, then slice and serve with a dollop of whipped coconut cream.
6. Scrumptious!

Old-Fashioned Molasses Candy

Yields: 1 (9-inch) pan

Ingredients:

2 cups rapadura

1 cup molasses

1 cup chopped nuts
(pecans, walnuts, or
almonds work well)

1 tablespoon organic butter

1 tablespoon organic apple
cider vinegar

$\frac{1}{8}$ teaspoon baking soda

Directions:

1. Combine the rapadura, molasses, butter, and apple cider vinegar in a large, heavy-bottomed saucepan, and cook until you have a syrup that will form a hard ball when dropped in cold water (265°F on a candy thermometer).

2. Remove the pan from the heat, add the baking soda, and stir well.

3. Stir in the nuts and pour the mixture into a buttered pan.

4. Cut into squares as it cools.

5. Try not to eat it all at once!

Homemade Gingerbread

Yields: 12 Servings

Ingredients:

2/3 cup milk
1/4 cup molasses
1/4 cup pure maple syrup
1/3 cup carrot juice
1 tablespoon organic apple
    cider vinegar
2 tablespoons melted coconut
    oil
2 tablespoons ground flaxseed
    meal

cup spelt flour
1 teaspoon baking soda
1/4 teaspoon salt
1 1/2 teaspoons powdered ginger
1 1/2 teaspoons cinnamon
1/2 teaspoon allspice
1/4 rapadura

Directions:

1. Preheat oven to 400 °F. and grease an 8 x 8-inch baking pan.
2. In a large mixing bowl, whisk together all the liquid ingredients and the flax seed meal. Let sit for at least 5 minutes.

3. In a separate mixing bowl, stir together all the remaining ingredients.
4. Pour the wet mixture into dry, and stir until they are evenly combined. Do not over mix.
5. Pour the combined mixture into the pan and bake 25 minutes.
6. Remove the gingerbread from the oven and let it sit for 20 minutes to achieve the correct texture and cool down.
7. Slice.
8. Gobble it up!

Apple Pie

Yields: 2 to 4 Portions

Ingredients:

For the Crust:

1 cup spelt flour

¼ teaspoon salt

4 tablespoons cold unsalted
butter, diced

¼ teaspoon organic apple cider
vinegar

3–4 tablespoons cold water

For the Filling:

2 apples

¾ teaspoon orange zest

⅛ teaspoon allspice

¼ teaspoon cinnamon

¼ cup rapadura

2 teaspoons milk, for brushing
on crust

Directions:

1. Crust: Stir together the salt and the flour in a medium bowl.

2. Now add the cold, diced butter, blending it using two knives. When the butter pieces are the size of peas, squeeze the dough using your hands. When you are able to form a clump, place the dough in a bowl and refrigerate for ten minutes.

3. Remove the dough after ten minutes, add the apple cider vinegar and two tablespoons of cold water. Stir with a fork, adding more water as required. Do not add more than five tablespoons of water.

4. Flatten the dough into a disk and wrap it in plastic, refrigerate for thirty minutes.

5. Preheat your oven to 425 °F. Have a six to seven inch metal pie tin ready to use.

6. Prepare the apples by peeling and slicing them thinly, then cut the slices in half. Add the apples to a bowl with the rapadura, allspice, cinnamon, and the zest and toss together.

7. Using a lightly floured surface, divide the dough in two. One portion should be slightly bigger than the other (for the base).

8. Roll the larger portion for the base into a circle 1 inch bigger than the pie pan and then gently fit it into the pan. Take care not to stretch the dough.

9. Roll the smaller portion into a circle the same size as the pie pan. Set it aside.

10. Add the apple filling to the pie pan and crust. Pat it down firmly to remove any air gaps.

11. Lay the set-aside pie crust over the top of the apple filling and pinch the two seams together decoratively. Cut two slits in the middle of the crust for ventilation. Brush the pie with milk and sprinkle some sugar over the top.

12. Bake for twenty minutes at 425 °F , then lower the temperature to 350°F and bake for a further fifteen to twenty minutes. The filling should be bubbling.

13. Remove from the oven to cool for two hours prior to serving.

14. A good old faithful classic!

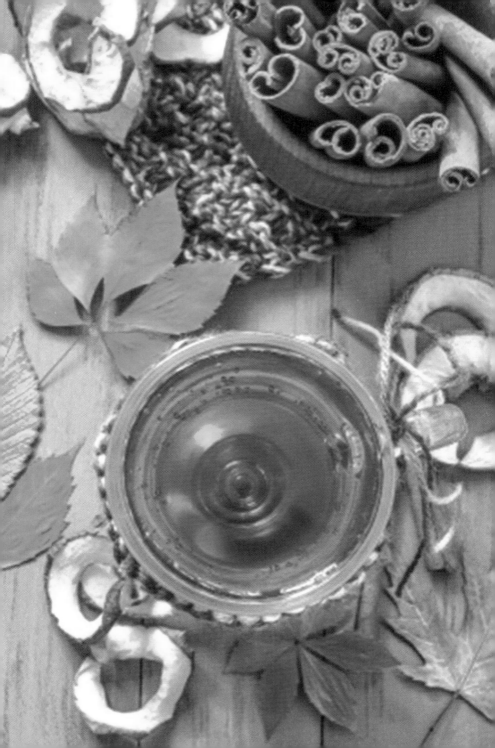

Healthy Drinks

Basic Apple Cider Vinegar Drink

Yields: 1 cup (250ml)

Mix 1 tablespoon of organic apple cider vinegar into 1 cup of warm purified water.

Optional: Sweeten with ½ teaspoon of raw organic honey if desired.

Healthy After Dinner Cordial

If you're looking for a more nutritious end to an elegant meal than an alcoholic beverage, try making a delicious fruit and vinegar cordial. Meld the apple flavors in apple cider vinegar with other fruits to get a beverage with an after-dinner glow that's truly good for you.

Start with any one of a variety of fruits, such as peaches, strawberries, cherries, blueberries, or black raspberries. Sterilize a quart canning jar and add 1 cup of one or more of the fruits listed above. Add 2 tablespoons of raw organic honey and cover with 2 cups of apple cider vinegar. Top with a canning lid and let it stand in a dark place for about two weeks. Strain off the liquid and serve in small cordial glasses with some crushed ice. Refreshing and tasty!

Special Detox Drink

The flavor of this detox drink may surprise you, but keep going. It's incredibly cleansing and good for you.

Yields: 1 cup (250ml)

Ingredients:

1 cup warm or room temperature filtered water

2 tablespoons organic apple cider vinegar

2 tablespoons lemon juice

1 teaspoon cinnamon, ground

1 teaspoon raw honey

Pinch of cayenne pepper, or to taste

Directions:

1. Mix all ingredients together in a large glass.
2. Drink immediately.

Green Machine

Yields: about 4 cups

Ingredients:

3 celery stalks
4 kale leaves
1 cup baby spinach leaves
3 lemons, peeled and chopped
1 ½ cups coconut water
¼ cup cilantro

1 tablespoon flax seeds
1 tablespoon organic apple
    cider vinegar
1 teaspoon coconut oil
Honey to taste (optional)

Directions:

1. Add the ingredients to your food processor and blend to your desired consistency.
2. Store in the fridge and consume within 24 hours.

Berry Blast Smoothie

Yields: 2 servings

Ingredients:

3 cups mixed berries, use a combination of blackberries, blueberries, raspberries and strawberries

1 cup almond milk

1 banana

1 tablespoon organic apple cider vinegar

Honey to taste (optional)

Ice cubes, as needed

Directions:

1. Blend it up.
2. Drink it down.
3. Yum!

Apple Cider Detoxer

Yields: about 2 ½ cups

Ingredients:

2 cups water

½ cup unsweetened apple juice

1 tablespoon organic apple
cider vinegar

1 teaspoon honey, or to taste

½ teaspoon ground ginger

½ teaspoon cinnamon

Directions:

1. Whisk all the ingredients together in a big jug.
2. Serve chilled.

The Headache Reliever

Yields: 1 serving

Ingredients:

2 cups water

2 tablespoons organic apple
cider vinegar

1 tablespoon cinnamon

1 tablespoon lemon juice

Directions:

1. Stir all the ingredients together and drink immediately.
2. You should feel relief within half an hour.

Berry Syrup

Yields: about 2 cups

Ingredients:

2 cups berries of your choice (raspberries, strawberries, blackberries work well)

½ cup raw honey

½ cup organic apple cider vinegar

2 tablespoons lemon juice

Directions:

1. Place the berries, lemon juice, and apple cider vinegar into a saucepan and bring to a boil over a medium heat.
2. Now transfer it to a glass jar and allow it to cool.
3. Once cool, cover it and allow it to sit for 24 hours at room temperature.
4. The next day, strain the liquid out into a saucepan and discard the berries.
5. Heat up the liquid and add the honey, allowing it to simmer for a few minutes until the honey is completely dissolved.
6. Remove from the heat and allow to cool down, then store in the fridge.
7. To serve: mix 25ml of berry syrup with 250 ml water or soda.
8. A taste sensation!

Tangy and Spicy Grape Juice

Yields: about 4 cups

Ingredients:

4 cups organic grape juice
Juice of 1 lemon
1 tablespoon organic apple
    cider vinegar

2 teaspoons cinnamon
1 teaspoon ground cloves

Directions:

1. Add the ingredients to a saucepan and bring it to a boil, then reduce the heat and allow to simmer for 5 minutes or until all the spices are well combined.
2. Turn off the heat and allow the mixture to come to room temperature.
3. Store in an airtight container in the fridge for up to 2 weeks.
4. Drink as is when desired.
5. Delicious!

Gingerbread Sipper

Yields: about 5 cups

Ingredients:

1 cup organic apple cider
vinegar
½ cup organic molasses
3 ½ cups water

3 teaspoons ground ginger
½ teaspoon nutmeg
½ teaspoon cinnamon

Directions:

1. Whisk all the ingredients together vigorously until combined properly.
2. Pour and serve.
3. Unusual and very tasty!

Citrus Blast

Yields: 1 serving

Ingredients:

1 ½ cups water

½ cup freshly squeezed orange juice

2 tablespoons organic apple cider vinegar

2 tablespoons honey, or to taste

2 tablespoons lime juice

Directions:

1. Place all the ingredients into an airtight jar.
2. Close the lid and shake vigorously until they are properly combined.
3. Pour and drink!

Cranberry Cooler

Yields: about 1 ½ cups

Ingredients:

1 ½ cups water
¼ cup fresh cranberries,
    crushed
4 tablespoons cranberry juice

2 tablespoons organic apple
    cider vinegar
1 tablespoon honey, optional

Directions:

1. Place the crushed cranberries into a large jug.
2. Add the rest of the ingredients and stir to combine.
3. Set into the fridge to chill.
4. Pour and serve.
5. Enjoy!

Virgin Bloody Mary

Yields: about 2 cups

Ingredients:

2 cups fresh tomato juice

2 tablespoons organic apple
    cider vinegar

Salt and pepper to taste

Hot sauce to taste, optional

1 celery stalk for serving

Directions:

1. Place all the ingredients into a large glass and stir together with the celery stalk.
2. Sip and relax!

The Pink Panther

Yields: about 1 ½ cups

Ingredients:

1 ½ cups freshly squeezed
    pink grapefruit juice
2 tablespoons honey, or to taste

2 tablespoons organic apple
    cider vinegar

Directions:

1. Mix it up.
2. Drink it down.
3. Feel the goodness!

Apple Cider Go-Go Juice

This juice will hold in the fridge for weeks if sealed properly so you can make large batches in advance to always have a pick me up on hand.

Yields: about 2½ cups

Ingredients:

2 cups water

½ cup organic apple cider vinegar

½ cup organic pomegranate juice, or fruit juice of your choice

2 tablespoons lemon juice

1 tablespoon honey, or to taste

1 teaspoon cinnamon

Directions:

1. Place all the ingredients in a jug with lots of ice and stir.
2. Store in the fridge and drink as desired.
3. Yum!

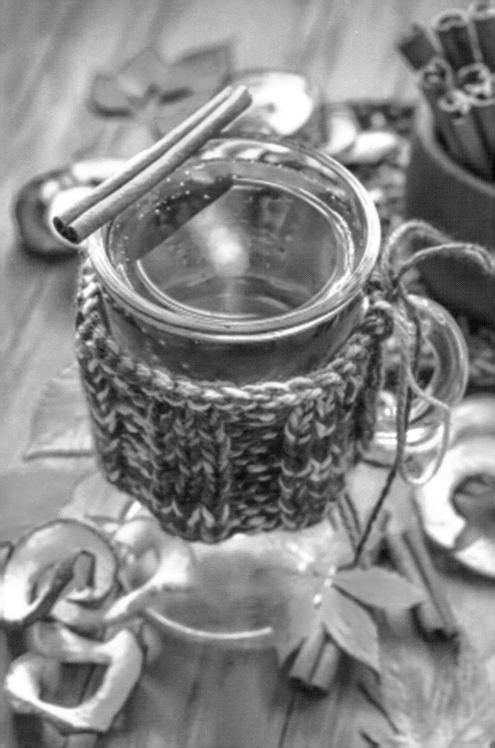

Conclusion

Apple cider vinegar truly is a magical elixir. There can be no downside to including it in your daily diet. So welcome health, beauty, and vitality into your life with as little as a tablespoon of this amazing liquid a day. There is no part of your body that is excluded from enjoying the miraculous benefits of apple cider vinegar, literally from top to toe, inside and outside; your body can enjoy something positive when you use it regularly.

So don't waste another minute—welcome apple cider vinegar into your life today! You won't regret it!

Index